Pennsylvania Ambulatory Surgery Center Certification and Licensure Regulations

A Guide to the Certification and Licensure Regulations Governing Free-Standing ASCs in Pennsylvania

2017 Edition

John J. Goehle, MBA, CASC, CPA
Chief Operating Officer
Ambulatory Healthcare Strategies, LLC

Published by:
Eden Group Development, Inc.
Spencerport, New York

Disclaimer:

This book is an educational and operational tool and is not intended to be a comprehensive resource for all rules, regulations and standards that an Ambulatory Surgery Center must meet. The author and publisher cannot accept any responsibility for errors or omissions or for any consequences from application of the information in this book and make no representations, warranties, express or implied, with respect to the contents of this book. The information in this book should not be considered as, nor does it constitute legal advice or opinion. When reviewing specific situations involving legal and regulatory issues, attorneys and other professionals should be consulted.

The author and publisher have exerted every effort to ensure that the information set forth in the text is current and accurate. However, in view of the ongoing changes in the ASC industry, changes in governmental regulations and the constant change in medical technology, the reader is urged to consult with qualified legal and ASC consultants for professional advice. The information contained in this book was gathered from publicly available information and references to the source are provided for the reader to review. Note that public records are not always updated in a timely manner and the reader should be careful to obtain and read information about recent changes to rules and regulations. The author and publisher have no responsibility for the accuracy of web site references in this book or the persistence of those web sites into the future.

Neither the author nor the publisher is affiliated with the State of Pennsylvania or the Centers for Medicare and Medicaid Services (CMS) in any way. The State of Pennsylvania and CMS assume no liability for the content of this book.

V2017-090217

Other Books by John J. Goehle

Published by HC Pro

Financial Management Made Easy – Strategies for Ambulatory Surgery Centers

APCs for ASCs – Strategies for Success under the New Payment System

Published by Eden Group Development

The Survey Guide for ASCs - A Guide to the Conditions for Coverage & Interpretive Guidelines for Ambulatory Surgery Centers

Ambulatory Surgery Center Governance - A Guide for Ambulatory Surgery Center Owners & Governing Body Members

Medicare Regulations & Payment Policy for Ambulatory Surgery Centers

Selected Federal and State Rules, Regulations & Standards for ASCs

Table of Contents

Ambulatory Surgery Centers in Pennsylvania must be certified by CMS as an ambulatory surgical facility to bill for Medicare services. In addition all ASCs in Pennsylvania must be licensed by the state.

This book is designed to be a handy summary both the Medicare Conditions for Coverage for Ambulatory Surgery Centers and the Pennsylvania licensing regulations.

The regulations included in this book are from publically available sources and based on information from July 2017.

It is important to check frequently for any changes to these regulations.

Medicare defines an Ambulatory Surgery Center as a "distinct entity that operates exclusively for the purpose of providing surgical services to patients not requiring hospitalization and in which the expected duration of services would not exceed 24 hours following an admission."

To become an ASC and bill the Medicare program and most other insurances, you must comply with the regulations established by CMS, as well as any state licensure requirements. In most states, you must be Medicare Certified to become licensed as an ASC within that state, even if you do not intend to take care of Medicare or Medicaid patients.

The Conditions for Coverage, issued by the Centers for Medicare and Medicaid Services (CMS) are the federal regulations that ASCs must meet to participate in the Medicare program and to obtain Medicare Certification.

These conditions (which include "standards" associated with each "condition") are updated periodically by CMS and those updates are published in the federal register. The conditions for coverage are broken into seven sections. This book contains an overview, a convenient index, and the complete text of the Conditions for Coverage.

Interpretive Guidelines for the Conditions for Coverage

The Centers for Medicare and Medicaid Services (CMS) provides guidance to State Surveyors regarding the interpretation of the Conditions for Coverage.

Revised guidance is posted periodically on the CMS website and the reader should check periodically for any updates. The web address for these updates is:

http://www.cms.gov/Medicare/Provider-Enrollment-and-Certification/SurveyCertificationGenInfo/Policy-and-Memos-to-States-and-Regions.html

When you load the site in your browser, you will want to search for "ASC" to bring up only Ambulatory Surgical Center Guidance.

It is highly recommended that ASCs review the guidelines and alerts as they provide an excellent summary of the rationale of the conditions and the accepted interpretation of their meaning. The clarifications are of particular importance given the focus survey teams tend to have on these issues.

The author publishes a companion to this book - The Survey Guide for ASCs - A Guide to the CMS Conditions for Coverage & Interpretive Guidelines for Ambulatory Surgery Centers which is available at Amazon or through the publisher's web site at www.reg-books.com.

Original Source Documentation

CMS maintains a web site that provides copies of the proposed and final rules as well as links to useful and updated information about the conditions:

http://www.cms.hhs.gov/CFCsAndCoPs/16_ASC.asp

The actual Conditions for Coverage are available through the Electronic Code of Federal Regulations Web Site (www.ecfr.gpoaccess.gov). The code is available through the following link and is reproduced in this book in its entirety.

http://www.ecfr.gov/cgi-bin/text-idx?c=ecfr&rgn=div5&view=text&node=42:3.0.1.1.3&idno=42

Note that the Conditions for Coverage are not the only rules and regulations that an ASC must follow to maintain Medicare certification and State licensure. ASC administrators should consult their state laws for state-specific requirements. Also note that the Conditions for Coverage refer extensively to the Life Safety Code published by the National Fire Protection Association (NFPA). ASCs should have a copy of the applicable Life Safety Code for their facility – which is available from their web site at:

http://nfpa.org

Lastly, please remember to consult attorneys with a thorough understanding of the ASC industry prior to making important decisions regarding your ASC. No single online or written resource can provide you with the up to date regulatory guidance that you receive from a knowledgeable attorney.

Introduction

This section contains the complete conditions for coverage as contained in the Federal Register. See Part III for the interpretation of these conditions. Note that Part III is broken down by Subpart and Chapter just as the conditions for coverage contained herein.

The Medicare Conditions for Coverage for ASCs

Per the Federal Register as of June 22, 2017

Authority: Secs. 1102 and 1871 of the Social Security Act (42 U.S.C. 1302 and 1395hh).

Source: 47 FR 34094, Aug. 5, 1982, unless otherwise noted.

Subpart A — General Provisions and Definitions

§416.1 Basis and scope.

(a) Statutory basis. (1) Section 1832(a)(2)(F)(i) of the Act provides for Medicare Part B coverage of facility services furnished in connection with surgical procedures specified by the Secretary under section 1833(i)(1) of the Act.

(2) Section 1833(i)(1)(A) of the Act requires the Secretary to specify the surgical procedures that can be performed safely on an ambulatory basis in an ambulatory surgical center.

(3) Sections 1833(i)(2)(A) and (D) and 1833(a)(1)(G) of the Act specify the amounts to be paid for facility services furnished in

connection with the specified surgical procedures when they are performed in an ASC.

(4) Section 1833(i)(2)(C) of the Act provides that if the Secretary has not updated amounts for ASC facility services furnished during a fiscal year through 2005 or a calendar year beginning with 2006, the amounts shall be increased by the percentage increase in the Consumer Price Index for all urban consumers as estimated by the Secretary for the 12-month period ending with the midpoint of the year involved, except that, in fiscal year 2005, the last quarter of calendar year 2005, and each of the calendar years 2006 through 2009, the increase shall be zero percent.

(5) Section 1833(i)(2)(E) of the Act provides that, with respect to surgical procedures furnished on or after January 1, 2007, and before the effective date of the implementation of a revised payment system, the payment amount shall be the lesser of the ASC payment rate established under section 1833(i)(2)(A) of the Act or the prospective payment rate for hospital outpatient department services established under section 1833(t)(3)(D) of the Act. The lesser payment amount shall be determined prior to application of any geographic adjustment.

(b) Scope. This part sets forth—

(1) The conditions that an ASC must meet in order to participate in the Medicare program;

(2) The scope of covered services; and

(3) The conditions for Medicare payment for facility services.

[56 FR 8843, Mar. 1, 1991; 56 FR 23022, May 20, 1991, as amended at 71 FR 68226, Nov. 24, 2006]

§416.2 Definitions.

As used in this part:

Ambulatory surgical center or ASC means any distinct entity that operates exclusively for the purpose of providing surgical services to patients not requiring hospitalization and in which the expected duration of services would not exceed 24 hours following an admission. The entity must have an agreement with CMS to participate in Medicare as an ASC, and must meet the conditions set forth in subparts B and C of this part.

ASC services means, for the period before January 1, 2008, facility services that are furnished in an ASC, and beginning January 1, 2008, means the combined facility services and covered ancillary services that are furnished in an ASC in connection with covered surgical procedures.

Covered ancillary services means items and services that are integral to a covered surgical procedure performed in an ASC as provided in §416.164(b), for which payment may be made under §416.171 in addition to the payment for the facility services.

Covered surgical procedures means those surgical procedures furnished before January 1, 2008, that meet the criteria specified in §416.65 and those surgical procedures furnished on or after January 1, 2008, that meet the criteria specified in §416.166.

Facility services means for the period before January 1, 2008, services that are furnished in connection with covered surgical procedures performed in an ASC, and beginning January 1, 2008, means services that are furnished in connection with covered surgical procedures performed in an ASC as provided in §416.164(a) for which payment is included in the ASC payment established under §416.171 for the covered surgical procedure.

[56 FR 8843, Mar. 1, 1991; 56 FR 23022, May 20, 1991, as amended at 71 FR 68226, Nov. 24, 2006; 72 FR 42544, Aug. 2, 2007; 73 FR 68811, Nov. 18, 2008]

Subpart B—General Conditions and Requirements

§416.25 Basic requirements.

Participation as an ASC is limited to facilities that—

(a) Meet the definition in §416.2; and

(b) Have in effect an agreement obtained in accordance with this subpart.

[56 FR 8843, Mar. 1, 1991]

§416.26 Qualifying for an agreement.

(a) Deemed compliance. CMS may deem an ASC to be in compliance with any or all of the conditions set forth in subpart C of this part if—

(1) The ASC is accredited by a national accrediting body, or licensed by a State agency, that CMS determines provides reasonable assurance that the conditions are met;

(2) In the case of deemed status through accreditation by a national accrediting body, where State law requires licensure, the ASC complies with State licensure requirements; and

(3) The ASC authorizes the release to CMS, of the findings of the accreditation survey.

(b) Survey of ASCs. (1) Unless CMS deems the ASC to be in compliance with the conditions set forth in subpart C of this part, the State survey agency must survey the facility to ascertain compliance with those conditions, and report its findings to CMS.

(2) CMS surveys deemed ASCs on a sample basis as part of CMS's validation process.

(c) Acceptance of the ASC as qualified to furnish ambulatory surgical services. If CMS determines, after reviewing the survey agency recommendation and other evidence relating to the qualification of the ASC, that the facility meets the requirements of this part, it sends to the ASC—

(1) Written notice of the determination; and

(2) Two copies of the ASC agreement.

(d) Filing of agreement by the ASC. If the ASC wishes to participate in the program, it must—

(1) Have both copies of the ASC agreement signed by its authorized representative; and

(2) File them with CMS.

(e) Acceptance by CMS. If CMS accepts the agreement filed by the ASC, returns to the ASC one copy of the agreement, with a notice of acceptance specifying the effective date.

(f) Appeal rights. If CMS refuses to enter into an agreement or if CMS terminates an agreement, the ASC is entitled to a hearing in accordance with part 498 of this chapter.

[56 FR 8843, Mar. 1, 1991]

§416.30   Terms of agreement with CMS.

As part of the agreement under §416.26 the ASC must agree to the following:

(a) Compliance with coverage conditions. The ASC agrees to meet the conditions for coverage specified in subpart C of this part and to report promptly to CMS any failure to do so.

(b) Limitation on charges to beneficiaries. The ASC agrees to charge the beneficiary or any other person only the applicable deductible and coinsurance amounts for facility services for which the beneficiary—

For facility services furnished before July 1987, the ASC had to agree to make no charge to the beneficiary, since those services were not subject to the part B deductible and coinsurance provisions.

(1) Is entitled to have payment made on his or her behalf under this part; or

(2) Would have been so entitled if the ASC had filed a request for payment in accordance with §410.165 of this chapter.

(c) Refunds to beneficiaries. (1) The ASC agrees to refund as promptly as possible any money incorrectly collected from beneficiaries or from someone on their behalf.

(2) As used in this section, money incorrectly collected means sums collected in excess of those specified in paragraph (b) of this section. It includes amounts collected for a period of time when the beneficiary was believed not to be entitled to Medicare benefits if—

(i) The beneficiary is later determined to have been entitled to Medicare benefits; and

(ii) The beneficiary's entitlement period falls within the time the ASC's agreement with CMS is in effect.

(d) Furnishing information. The ASC agrees to furnish to CMS, if requested, information necessary to establish payment rates specified in §§416.120-416.130 in the form and manner that CMS requires.

(e) Acceptance of assignment. The ASC agrees to accept assignment for all facility services furnished in connection with covered surgical procedures. For purposes of this section, assignment means an assignment under §424.55 of this chapter of the right to receive payment under Medicare Part B and payment under §424.64 of this chapter (when an individual dies before assigning the claim).

(f) ASCs operated by a hospital. In an ASC operated by a hospital—

(1) The agreement is made effective on the first day of the next Medicare cost reporting period of the hospital that operates the ASC; and

(2) The ASC participates and is paid only as an ASC.

(3) Costs for the ASC are treated as a non-reimbursable cost center on the hospital's cost report.

(g) Additional provisions. The agreement may contain any additional provisions that CMS finds necessary or desirable for the efficient and effective administration of the Medicare program.

[47 FR 34094, Aug. 5, 1982, as amended at 51 FR 41351, Nov. 14, 1986; 56 FR 8844, Mar. 1, 1991; 74 FR 60680, Nov. 20, 2009]

§416.35 Termination of agreement.

(a) Termination by the ASC—(1) Notice to CMS. An ASC that wishes to terminate its agreement must send CMS written notice of its intent.

(2) Date of termination. The notice may state the intended date of termination which must be the first day of a calendar month.

(i) If the notice does not specify a date, or the date is not acceptable to CMS, CMS may set a date that will not be more than 6 months from the date on the ASC's notice of intent.

(ii) CMS may accept a termination date that is less than 6 months after the date on the ASC's notice if it determines that to do so would not unduly disrupt services to the community or otherwise interfere with the effective and efficient administration of the Medicare program.

(3) Voluntary termination. If an ASC ceases to furnish services to the community, that shall be deemed to be a voluntary termination of the agreement by the ASC, effective on the last day of business with Medicare beneficiaries.

(b) Termination by CMS—(1) Cause for termination. CMS may terminate an agreement if it determines that the ASC—

(i) No longer meets the conditions for coverage as specified under §416.26; or

(ii) Is not in substantial compliance with the provisions of the agreement, the requirements of this subpart, and other applicable regulations of subchapter B of this chapter, or any applicable provisions of title XVIII of the Act.

(2) Notice of termination. CMS sends notice of termination to the ASC at least 15 days before the effective date stated in the notice.

(3) Appeal by the ASC. An ASC may appeal the termination of its agreement in accordance with the provisions set forth in part 498 of this chapter.

(c) Effect of termination. Payment is not available for ASC services furnished on or after the effective date of termination.

(d) Notice to the public. Prompt notice of the date and effect of termination is given to the public, through publication in local newspapers by—

(1) The ASC, after CMS has approved or set a termination date; or

(2) CMS, when it has terminated the agreement.

(e) Conditions for reinstatement after termination of agreement by CMS. When an agreement with an ASC is terminated by CMS, the ASC may not file another agreement to participate in the Medicare program unless CMS—

(1) Finds that the reason for the termination of the prior agreement has been removed; and

(2) Is assured that the reason for the termination will not recur.

[47 FR 34094, Aug. 5, 1982, as amended at 52 FR 22454, June 12, 1987; 56 FR 8844, Mar. 1, 1991; 61 FR 40347, Aug. 2, 1996]

Subpart C—Specific Conditions for Coverage

§416.40   Condition for coverage—Compliance with State licensure law.

The ASC must comply with State licensure requirements.

§416.41   Condition for coverage—Governing body and management.

The ASC must have a governing body that assumes full legal responsibility for determining, implementing, and monitoring policies governing the ASC's total operation. The governing body has oversight and accountability for the quality assessment and performance improvement program, ensures that facility policies and programs are administered so as to provide quality health care in a safe environment, and develops and maintains a disaster preparedness plan.

(a) Standard: Contract services. When services are provided through a contract with an outside resource, the ASC must assure that these services are provided in a safe and effective manner.

(b) Standard: Hospitalization. (1) The ASC must have an effective procedure for the immediate transfer, to a hospital, of patients requiring emergency medical care beyond the capabilities of the ASC.

(2) This hospital must be a local, Medicare-participating hospital or a local, nonparticipating hospital that meets the requirements for payment for emergency services under §482.2 of this chapter.

(3) The ASC must—

(i) Have a written transfer agreement with a hospital that meets the requirements of paragraph (b)(2) of this section; or

(ii) Ensure that all physicians performing surgery in the ASC have admitting privileges at a hospital that meets the requirements of paragraph (b)(2) of this section.

[73 FR 68811, Nov. 18, 2008, as amended at 81 FR 64022, Sept. 16, 2016]

§416.42   Condition for coverage—Surgical services.

Surgical procedures must be performed in a safe manner by qualified physicians who have been granted clinical privileges by the governing body of the ASC in accordance with approved policies and procedures of the ASC.

(a) Standard: Anesthetic risk and evaluation. (1) A physician must examine the patient immediately before surgery to evaluate the risk of anesthesia and of the procedure to be performed.

(2) Before discharge from the ASC, each patient must be evaluated by a physician or by an anesthetist as defined at §410.69(b) of this chapter, in accordance with applicable State health and safety laws, standards of practice, and ASC policy, for proper anesthesia recovery.

(b) Standard: Administration of anesthesia. Anesthetics must be administered by only—

(1) A qualified anesthesiologist; or

(2) A physician qualified to administer anesthesia, a certified registered nurse anesthetist (CRNA), or an anesthesiologist's assistant as defined in §410.69(b) of this chapter, or a supervised trainee in an approved educational program. In those cases in which a non-physician administers the anesthesia, unless exempted in accordance with paragraph (c) of this section, the anesthetist must be under the supervision of the operating physician, and in the case of an anesthesiologist's assistant, under the supervision of an anesthesiologist.

(c) Standard: State exemption. (1) An ASC may be exempted from the requirement for physician supervision of CRNAs as described in paragraph (b)(2) of this section, if the State in which the ASC is located submits a letter to CMS signed by the Governor, following consultation with the State's Boards of Medicine and Nursing, requesting exemption from physician supervision of CRNAs. The letter from the Governor must attest that he or she has consulted with State Boards of Medicine and Nursing about issues related to access to and the quality of anesthesia services in the State and has concluded that it is in the best interests of the State's citizens to opt-out of the current physician supervision requirement, and that the opt-out is consistent with State law.

(2) The request for exemption and recognition of State laws and the withdrawal of the request may be submitted at any time, and are effective upon submission.

[57 FR 33899, July 31, 1992, as amended at 66 FR 56768, Nov. 13, 2001; 73 FR 68812, Nov. 18, 2008; 79 FR 27153, May 12, 2014]

§416.43 Conditions for coverage—Quality assessment and performance improvement.

The ASC must develop, implement and maintain an ongoing, data-driven quality assessment and performance improvement (QAPI) program.

(a) Standard: Program scope. (1) The program must include, but not be limited to, an ongoing program that demonstrates measurable improvement in patient health outcomes, and improves patient safety by using quality indicators or performance measures associated with improved health outcomes and by the identification and reduction of medical errors.

(2) The ASC must measure, analyze, and track quality indicators, adverse patient events, infection control and other aspects of performance that includes care and services furnished in the ASC.

(b) Standard: Program data. (1) The program must incorporate quality indicator data, including patient care and other relevant data regarding services furnished in the ASC.

(2) The ASC must use the data collected to—

(i) Monitor the effectiveness and safety of its services, and quality of its care.

(ii) Identify opportunities that could lead to improvements and changes in its patient care.

(c) Standard: Program activities. (1) The ASC must set priorities for its performance improvement activities that—

(i) Focus on high risk, high volume, and problem-prone areas.

(ii) Consider incidence, prevalence, and severity of problems in those areas.

(iii) Affect health outcomes, patient safety, and quality of care.

(2) Performance improvement activities must track adverse patient events, examine their causes, implement improvements, and ensure that improvements are sustained over time.

(3) The ASC must implement preventive strategies throughout the facility targeting adverse patient events and ensure that all staff are familiar with these strategies.

(d) Standard: Performance improvement projects. (1) The number and scope of distinct improvement projects conducted annually must reflect the scope and complexity of the ASC's services and operations.

(2) The ASC must document the projects that are being conducted. The documentation, at a minimum, must include the reason(s) for implementing the project, and a description of the project's results.

(e) Standard: Governing body responsibilities. The governing body must ensure that the QAPI program—

(1) Is defined, implemented, and maintained by the ASC.

(2) Addresses the ASC's priorities and that all improvements are evaluated for effectiveness.

(3) Specifies data collection methods, frequency, and details.

(4) Clearly establishes its expectations for safety.

(5) Adequately allocates sufficient staff, time, information systems and training to implement the QAPI program.

[73 FR 68812, Nov. 18, 2008]

§416.44 Condition for coverage—Environment.

The ASC must have a safe and sanitary environment, properly constructed, equipped, and maintained to protect the health and safety of patients.

(a) Standard: Physical environment. The ASC must provide a functional and sanitary environment for the provision of surgical services.

(1) Each operating room must be designed and equipped so that the types of surgery conducted can be performed in a manner that protects the lives and assures the physical safety of all individuals in the area.

(2) The ASC must have a separate recovery room and waiting area.

(b) Standard: Safety from fire. (1) Except as otherwise provided in this section, the ASC must meet the provisions applicable to Ambulatory Health Care Occupancies, regardless of the number of patients served, and must proceed in accordance with the Life

Safety Code (NFPA 101 and Tentative Interim Amendments TIA 12-1, TIA 12-2, TIA 12-3, and TIA 12-4).

(2) In consideration of a recommendation by the State survey agency or Accrediting Organization or at the discretion of the Secretary, may waive, for periods deemed appropriate, specific provisions of the Life Safety Code, which would result in unreasonable hardship upon an ASC, but only if the waiver will not adversely affect the health and safety of the patients.

(3) The provisions of the Life Safety Code do not apply in a State if CMS finds that a fire and safety code imposed by State law adequately protects patients in an ASC.

(4) An ASC may place alcohol-based hand rub dispensers in its facility if the dispensers are installed in a manner that adequately protects against inappropriate access.

(5) When a sprinkler system is shut down for more than 10 hours, the ASC must:

(i) Evacuate the building or portion of the building affected by the system outage until the system is back in service, or

(ii) Establish a fire watch until the system is back in service.

(6) Beginning July 5, 2017, an ASC must be in compliance with Chapter 21.3.2.1, Doors to hazardous areas.

© Standard: Building Safety. Except as otherwise provided in this section, the ASC must meet the applicable provisions and must proceed in accordance with the 2012 edition of the Health Care Facilities Code (NFPA 99, and Tentative Interim Amendments TIA 12-2, TIA 12-3, TIA 12-4, TIA 12-5 and TIA 12-6).

(1) Chapters 7, 8, 12, and 13 of the adopted Health Care Facilities Code do not apply to an ASC.

(2) If application of the Health Care Facilities Code required under paragraph (c) of this section would result in unreasonable hardship for the ASC, CMS may waive specific provisions of the Health Care Facilities Code, but only if the waiver does not adversely affect the health and safety of patients.

(d) Standard: Emergency equipment. The ASC medical staff and governing body of the ASC coordinates, develops, and revises ASC policies and procedures to specify the types of emergency equipment required for use in the ASC's operating room. The equipment must meet the following requirements:

(1) Be immediately available for use during emergency situations.

(2) Be appropriate for the facility's patient population.

(3) Be maintained by appropriate personnel.

(e) Standard: Emergency personnel. Personnel trained in the use of emergency equipment and in cardiopulmonary resuscitation must be available whenever there is a patient in the ASC.

(f) The standards incorporated by reference in this section are approved for incorporation by reference by the Director of the Office of the Federal Register in accordance with 5 U.S.C. 552(a) and 1 CFR part 51. You may inspect a copy at the CMS Information Resource Center, 7500 Security Boulevard, Baltimore, MD or at the National Archives and Records Administration (NARA). For information on the availability of this material at NARA, call 202-741-6030, or go to:

http://www.archives.gov/federal_register/code_of_federal_regulati ons/ibr_locations.html. If any changes in this edition of the Code are incorporated by reference, CMS will publish a document in the FEDERAL REGISTER to announce the changes.

(1) National Fire Protection Association, 1 Batterymarch Park, Quincy, MA 02169, www.nfpa.org, 1.617.770.3000.

(i) NFPA 99, Standards for Health Care facilities Code of the National Fire Protection Association 99, 2012 edition, issued August 11, 2011.

(ii) TIA 12-2 to NFPA 99, issued August 11, 2011.

(iii) TIA 12-3 to NFPA 99, issued August 9, 2012.

(iv) TIA 12-4 to NFPA 99, issued March 7, 2013.

(v) TIA 12-5 to NFPA 99, issued August 1, 2013.

(vi) TIA 12-6 to NFPA 99, issued March 3, 2014.

(vii) NFPA 101, Life Safety Code, 2012 edition, issued August 11, 2011;

(viii) TIA 12-1 to NFPA 101, issued August 11, 2011.

(ix) TIA 12-2 to NFPA 101, issued October 30, 2012.

(x) TIA 12-3 to NFPA 101, issued October 22, 2013.

(xi) TIA 12-4 to NFPA 101, issued October 22, 2013.

(2) [Reserved]

[47 FR 34094, Aug. 5, 1982, amended at 53 FR 11508, Apr. 7, 1988; 54 FR 4026, Jan. 27, 1989; 68 FR 1385, Jan. 10, 2003; 69 FR 18803, Apr. 9, 2004; 70 FR 15237, Mar. 25, 2005; 71 FR 55339, Sept. 22, 2006; 77 FR 29030, May 16, 2012; 81 FR 26896, May 4, 2016; 81 FR 42548, June 30, 2016]

§416.45 Condition for coverage—Medical staff.

The medical staff of the ASC must be accountable to the governing body.

(a) Standard: Membership and clinical privileges. Members of the medical staff must be legally and professionally qualified for the positions to which they are appointed and for the performance of privileges granted. The ASC grants privileges in accordance with recommendations from qualified medical personnel.

(b) Standard: Reappraisals. Medical staff privileges must be periodically reappraised by the ASC. The scope of procedures performed in the ASC must be periodically reviewed and amended as appropriate.

(c) Standard: Other practitioners. If the ASC assigns patient care responsibilities to practitioners other than physicians, it must have established policies and procedures, approved by the governing body, for overseeing and evaluating their clinical activities.

§416.46 Condition for coverage—Nursing services.

The nursing services of the ASC must be directed and staffed to assure that the nursing needs of all patients are met.

(a) Standard: Organization and staffing. Patient care responsibilities must be delineated for all nursing service personnel. Nursing services must be provided in accordance with recognized standards of practice. There must be a registered nurse available for emergency treatment whenever there is a patient in the ASC.

(b) [Reserved]

§416.47 Condition for coverage—Medical records.

The ASC must maintain complete, comprehensive, and accurate medical records to ensure adequate patient care.

(a) Standard: Organization. The ASC must develop and maintain a system for the proper collection, storage, and use of patient records.

(b) Standard: Form and content of record. The ASC must maintain a medical record for each patient. Every record must be accurate, legible, and promptly completed. Medical records must include at least the following:

(1) Patient identification.

(2) Significant medical history and results of physical examination.

(3) Pre-operative diagnostic studies (entered before surgery), if performed.

(4) Findings and techniques of the operation, including a pathologist's report on all tissues removed during surgery, except those exempted by the governing body.

(5) Any allergies and abnormal drug reactions.

(6) Entries related to anesthesia administration.

(7) Documentation of properly executed informed patient consent.

(8) Discharge diagnosis.

§416.48 Condition for coverage—Pharmaceutical services.

The ASC must provide drugs and biologicals in a safe and effective manner, in accordance with accepted professional practice, and under the direction of an individual designated responsible for pharmaceutical services.

(a) Standard: Administration of drugs. Drugs must be prepared and administered according to established policies and acceptable standards of practice.

(1) Adverse reactions must be reported to the physician responsible for the patient and must be documented in the record.

(2) Blood and blood products must be administered by only physicians or registered nurses.

(3) Orders given orally for drugs and biologicals must be followed by a written order, signed by the prescribing physician.

(b) [Reserved]

§416.49   Condition for coverage—Laboratory and radiologic services.

(a) Standard: Laboratory services. If the ASC performs laboratory services, it must meet the requirements of part 493 of this chapter. If the ASC does not provide its own laboratory services, it must have procedures for obtaining routine and emergency laboratory services from a certified laboratory in accordance with part 493 of this chapter. The referral laboratory must be certified in the appropriate specialties and subspecialties of service to perform the referred tests in accordance with the requirements of Part 493 of this chapter.

(b) Standard: Radiologic services. (1) Radiologic services may only be provided when integral to procedures offered by the ASC and must meet the requirements specified in §482.26(b), (c)(2), and (d)(2) of this chapter.

(2) If radiologic services are utilized, the governing body must appoint an individual qualified in accordance with State law and ASC policies who is responsible for assuring all radiologic services are provided in accordance with the requirements of this section.

[73 FR 68812, Nov. 18, 2008, as amended at 79 FR 27153, May 12, 2014]

§416.50   Condition for coverage—Patient rights.

The ASC must inform the patient or the patient's representative or surrogate of the patient's rights and must protect and promote the exercise of these rights, as set forth in this section. The ASC must also post the written notice of patient rights in a place or places within the ASC likely to be noticed by patients waiting for treatment or by the patient's representative or surrogate, if applicable.

(a) Standard: Notice of Rights. An ASC must, prior to the start of the surgical procedure, provide the patient, the patient's representative, or the patient's surrogate with verbal and written notice of the patient's rights in a language and manner that ensures the patient, the representative, or the surrogate understand all of the patient's rights as set forth in this section. The ASC's notice of rights must include the address and telephone number of the State agency to which patients may report complaints, as well as the Web site for the Office of the Medicare Beneficiary Ombudsman.

(b) Standard: Disclosure of physician financial interest or ownership. The ASC must disclose, in accordance with Part 420 of this subchapter, and where applicable, provide a list of physicians who have financial interest or ownership in the ASC facility. Disclosure of information must be in writing.

(c) Standard: Advance directives. The ASC must comply with the following requirements:

(1) Provide the patient or, as appropriate, the patient's representative with written information concerning its policies on advance directives, including a description of applicable State health and safety laws and, if requested, official State advance directive forms.

(2) Inform the patient or, as appropriate, the patient's representative of the patient's right to make informed decisions regarding the patient's care.

(3) Document in a prominent part of the patient's current medical record, whether or not the individual has executed an advance directive.

(d) Standard: Submission and investigation of grievances. The ASC must establish a grievance procedure for documenting the existence, submission, investigation, and disposition of a patient's written or verbal grievance to the ASC. The following criteria must be met:

(1) All alleged violations/grievances relating, but not limited to, mistreatment, neglect, verbal, mental, sexual, or physical abuse, must be fully documented.

(2) All allegations must be immediately reported to a person in authority in the ASC.

(3) Only substantiated allegations must be reported to the State authority or the local authority, or both.

(4) The grievance process must specify timeframes for review of the grievance and the provisions of a response.

(5) The ASC, in responding to the grievance, must investigate all grievances made by a patient, the patient's representative, or the

patient's surrogate regarding treatment or care that is (or fails to be) furnished.

(6) The ASC must document how the grievance was addressed, as well as provide the patient, the patient's representative, or the patient's surrogate with written notice of its decision. The decision must contain the name of an ASC contact person, the steps taken to investigate the grievance, the result of the grievance process and the date the grievance process was completed.

(e) Standard: Exercise of rights and respect for property and person. (1) The patient has the right to the following:

(i) Be free from any act of discrimination or reprisal.

(ii) Voice grievances regarding treatment or care that is (or fails to be) provided.

(iii) Be fully informed about a treatment or procedure and the expected outcome before it is performed.

(2) If a patient is adjudged incompetent under applicable State laws by a court of proper jurisdiction, the rights of the patient are exercised by the person appointed under State law to act on the patient's behalf.

(3) If a State court has not adjudged a patient incompetent, any legal representative or surrogate designated by the patient in accordance with State law may exercise the patient's rights to the extent allowed by State law.

(f) Standard: Privacy and safety. The patient has the right to—

(1) Personal privacy.

(2) Receive care in a safe setting.

(3) Be free from all forms of abuse or harassment.

(g) Standard: Confidentiality of clinical records. The ASC must comply with the Department's rules for the privacy and security of individually identifiable health information, as specified at 45 CFR parts 160 and 164.

[73 FR 68812, Nov. 18, 2008, as amended at 76 FR 65889, Oct. 24, 2011]

§416.51 Conditions for coverage—Infection control.

The ASC must maintain an infection control program that seeks to minimize infections and communicable diseases.

(a) Standard: Sanitary environment. The ASC must provide a functional and sanitary environment for the provision of surgical services by adhering to professionally acceptable standards of practice.

(b) Standard: Infection control program. The ASC must maintain an ongoing program designed to prevent, control, and investigate infections and communicable diseases. In addition, the infection control and prevention program must include documentation that the ASC has considered, selected, and implemented nationally recognized infection control guidelines. The program is—

(1) Under the direction of a designated and qualified professional who has training in infection control;

(2) An integral part of the ASC's quality assessment and performance improvement program; and

(3) Responsible for providing a plan of action for preventing, identifying, and managing infections and communicable diseases

and for immediately implementing corrective and preventive measures that result in improvement.

[73 FR 68813, Nov. 18, 2008]
§416.52 Conditions for coverage—Patient admission, assessment and discharge.

The ASC must ensure each patient has the appropriate pre-surgical and post-surgical assessments completed and that all elements of the discharge requirements are completed.

(a) Standard: Admission and pre-surgical assessment. (1) Not more than 30 days before the date of the scheduled surgery, each patient must have a comprehensive medical history and physical assessment completed by a physician (as defined in section 1861(r) of the Act) or other qualified practitioner in accordance with applicable State health and safety laws, standards of practice, and ASC policy.

(2) Upon admission, each patient must have a pre-surgical assessment completed by a physician or other qualified practitioner in accordance with applicable State health and safety laws, standards of practice, and ASC policy that includes, at a minimum, an updated medical record entry documenting an examination for any changes in the patient's condition since completion of the most recently documented medical history and physical assessment, including documentation of any allergies to drugs and biologicals.

(3) The patient's medical history and physical assessment must be placed in the patient's medical record prior to the surgical procedure.

(b) Standard: Post-surgical assessment. (1) The patient's post-surgical condition must be assessed and documented in the medical record by a physician, other qualified practitioner, or a registered nurse with, at a minimum, post-operative care experience in accordance with applicable State health and safety laws, standards of practice, and ASC policy.

(2) Post-surgical needs must be addressed and included in the discharge notes.

(c) Standard: Discharge. The ASC must—

(1) Provide each patient with written discharge instructions and overnight supplies. When appropriate, make a follow-up appointment with the physician, and ensure that all patients are informed, either in advance of their surgical procedure or prior to leaving the ASC, of their prescriptions, post-operative instructions and physician contact information for follow-up care.

(2) Ensure each patient has a discharge order, signed by the physician who performed the surgery or procedure in accordance with applicable State health and safety laws, standards of practice, and ASC policy.

(3) Ensure all patients are discharged in the company of a responsible adult, except those patients exempted by the attending physician.

[73 FR 68813, Nov. 18, 2008]

§416.52 Conditions for coverage—Emergency preparedness.

The Ambulatory Surgical Center (ASC) must comply with all applicable Federal, State, and local emergency preparedness requirements. The ASC must establish and maintain an emergency preparedness program that meets the requirements of this section. The emergency preparedness program must include, but not be limited to, the following elements:

(a) Emergency plan. The ASC must develop and maintain an emergency preparedness plan that must be reviewed, and updated at least annually. The plan must do the following:

(1) Be based on and include a documented, facility-based and community-based risk assessment, utilizing an all-hazards approach.

(2) Include strategies for addressing emergency events identified by the risk assessment.

(3) Address patient population, including, but not limited to, the type of services the ASC has the ability to provide in an emergency; and continuity of operations, including delegations of authority and succession plans.

(4) Include a process for cooperation and collaboration with local, tribal, regional, State, and Federal emergency preparedness officals' efforts to maintain an integrated response during a disaster or emergency situation, including documentation of the ASC's efforts to contact such officials and, when applicable, of its participation in collaborative and cooperative planning efforts.

(b) Policies and procedures. The ASC must develop and implement emergency preparedness policies and procedures, based on the emergency plan set forth in paragraph (a) of this section, risk assessment at paragraph (a)(1) of this section, and the communication plan at paragraph (c) of this section. The policies and procedures must be reviewed and updated at least annually. At a minimum, the policies and procedures must address the following:

(1) A system to track the location of on-duty staff and sheltered patients in the ASC's care during an emergency. If on-duty staff or sheltered patients are relocated during the emergency, the ASC

must document the specific name and location of the receiving facility or other location.

(2) Safe evacuation from the ASC, which includes the following:

(i) Consideration of care and treatment needs of evacuees.

(ii) Staff responsibilities.

(iii) Transportation.

(iv) Identification of evacuation location(s).

(v) Primary and alternate means of communication with external sources of assistance.

(3) A means to shelter in place for patients, staff, and volunteers who remain in the ASC.

(4) A system of medical documentation that does the following:

(i) Preserves patient information.

(ii) Protects confidentiality of patient information.

(iii) Secures and maintains the availability of records.

(5) The use of volunteers in an emergency and other staffing strategies, including the process and role for integration of State and Federally designated health care professionals to address surge needs during an emergency.

(6) The role of the ASC under a waiver declared by the Secretary, in accordance with section 1135 of the Act, in the provision of care and treatment at an alternate care site identified by emergency management officials.

(c) Communication plan. The ASC must develop and maintain an emergency preparedness communication plan that complies with Federal, State, and local laws and must be reviewed and updated at least annually. The communication plan must include all of the following:

(1) Names and contact information for the following:

(i) Staff.

(ii) Entities providing services under arrangement.

(iii) Patients' physicians.

(iv) Volunteers.

(2) Contact information for the following:

(i) Federal, State, tribal, regional, and local emergency preparedness staff.

(ii) Other sources of assistance.

(3) Primary and alternate means for communicating with the following:

(i) ASC's staff.

(ii) Federal, State, tribal, regional, and local emergency management agencies.

(4) A method for sharing information and medical documentation for patients under the ASC's care, as necessary, with other health care providers to maintain continuity of care.

(5) A means, in the event of an evacuation, to release patient information as permitted under 45 CFR 164.510(b)(1)(ii).

(6) A means of providing information about the general condition and location of patients under the facility's care as permitted under 45 CFR 164.510(b)(4).

(7) A means of providing information about the ASC's needs, and its ability to provide assistance, to the authority having jurisdiction, the Incident Command Center, or designee.

(d) Training and testing. The ASC must develop and maintain an emergency preparedness training and testing program that is based on the emergency plan set forth in paragraph (a) of this section, risk assessment at paragraph (a)(1) of this section, policies and procedures at paragraph (b) of this section, and the communication plan at paragraph (c) of this section. The training and testing program must be reviewed and updated at least annually.

(1) Training program. The ASC must do all of the following:

(i) Initial training in emergency preparedness policies and procedures to all new and existing staff, individuals providing on-site services under arrangement, and volunteers, consistent with their expected roles.

(ii) Provide emergency preparedness training at least annually.

(iii) Maintain documentation of all emergency preparedness training.

(iv) Demonstrate staff knowledge of emergency procedures.

(2) Testing. The ASC must conduct exercises to test the emergency plan at least annually. The ASC must do the following:

(i) Participate in a full-scale exercise that is community-based or when a community-based exercise is not accessible, individual, facility-based. If the ASC experiences an actual natural or man-made emergency that requires activation of the emergency plan, the ASC is exempt -from engaging in a community-based or individual, facility-based full-scale exercise for 1 year following the onset of the actual event.

(ii) Conduct an additional exercise that may include, but is not limited to the following:

(A) a second full-scale exercise that is individual, facility-based.

(B) A tabletop exercise that includes a group discussion led by a facilitator, using narrated, clinically relevant emergency scenario, and a set of problem statements, directed messages, or prepared questions designed to challenge an emergency plan.

(iii) Analyze the ASC's response to and maintain documentation of all drills, tabletop exercises, and emergency events and revise the ASC's emergency plan, as needed.

(e) Integrated healthcare systems. If an ASC is part of a healthcare system consisting of multiple separately certified healthcare facilities that elects to have a unified and integrated emergency preparedness program, the ASC may choose to participate in the healthcare system's coordinated emergency preparedness program. If elected, the unified and integrated emergency preparedness program must—

(1) Demonstrate that each separately certified facility within the system actively participated in the development of the unified and integrated emergency preparedness program.

(2) Be developed and maintained in a manner that takes into account each separately certified facility's unique circumstances, patient populations, and services offered.

(3) Demonstrate that each separately certified facility is capable of actively using the unified and integrated emergency preparedness program and is in compliance.

(4) Include a unified and integrated emergency plan that meets the requirements of paragraphs (a)(2), (3), and (4) of this section. The unified and integrated emergency plan must also be based on and include the following:

(i) A documented community-based risk assessment, utilizing an all-hazards approach.

(ii) A documented individual facility-based risk assessment for each separately certified facility within the health system, utilizing an all-hazards approach.

(5) Include integrated policies and procedures that meet the requirements set forth in paragraph (b) of this section, a coordinated communication plan and training and testing programs that meet the requirements of paragraphs (c) and (d) of this section, respectively.

[81 FR 64022, Sept. 16, 2016]

Subpart D—Scope of Benefits for Services Furnished Before January 1, 2008

§416.60 General rules.

(a) The services payable under this part are facility services furnished to Medicare beneficiaries, by a participating facility, in connection with covered surgical procedures specified in §416.65.

(b) The surgical procedures, including all preoperative and post-operative services that are performed by a physician, are covered as physician services under part 410 of this chapter.

[56 FR 8844, Mar. 1, 1991]

§416.61 Scope of facility services.

(a) Included services. Facility services include, but are not limited to—

(1) Nursing, technician, and related services;

(2) Use of the facilities where the surgical procedures are performed;

(3) Drugs, biologicals, surgical dressings, supplies, splints, casts, and appliances and equipment directly related to the provision of surgical procedures;

(4) Diagnostic or therapeutic services or items directly related to the provision of a surgical procedure;

(5) Administrative, recordkeeping and housekeeping items and services; and

(6) Materials for anesthesia.

(7) Intra-ocular lenses (IOLs).

(8) Supervision of the services of an anesthetist by the operating surgeon.

(b) Excluded services. Facility services do not include items and services for which payment may be made under other provisions of part 405 of this chapter, such as physicians' services, laboratory, X-ray or diagnostic procedures (other than those directly related to performance of the surgical procedure), prosthetic devices (except IOLs), ambulance services, leg, arm, back and neck braces, artificial limbs, and durable medical equipment for use in the patient's home. In addition, they do not include anesthetist services furnished on or after January 1, 1989.

[56 FR 8844, Mar. 1, 1991, as amended at 57 FR 33899, July 31, 1992]

§416.65   Covered surgical procedures.

Effective for services furnished before January 1, 2008, covered surgical procedures are those procedures that meet the standards described in paragraphs (a) and (b) of this section and are included in the list published in accordance with paragraph (c) of this section.

(a) General standards. Covered surgical procedures are those surgical and other medical procedures that—

(1) Are commonly performed on an inpatient basis in hospitals, but may be safely performed in an ASC;

(2) Are not of a type that are commonly performed, or that may be safely performed, in physicians' offices;

(3) Are limited to those requiring a dedicated operating room (or suite), and generally requiring a post-operative recovery room or short-term (not overnight) convalescent room; and

(4) Are not otherwise excluded under §411.15 of this chapter.

(b) Specific standards. (1) Covered surgical procedures are limited to those that do not generally exceed—

(i) A total of 90 minutes operating time; and

(ii) A total of 4 hours recovery or convalescent time.

(2) If the covered surgical procedures require anesthesia, the anesthesia must be—

(i) Local or regional anesthesia; or

(ii) General anesthesia of 90 minutes or less duration.

(3) Covered surgical procedures may not be of a type that—

(i) Generally result in extensive blood loss;

(ii) Require major or prolonged invasion of body cavities;

(iii) Directly involve major blood vessels; or

(iv) Are generally emergency or life-threatening in nature.

(c) Publication of covered procedures. CMS will publish in the Federal Register a list of covered surgical procedures and revisions as appropriate.

[47 FR 34094, Aug. 5, 1982, as amended at 71 FR 68226, Nov. 24, 2006]

§416.75 Performance of listed surgical procedures on an inpatient hospital basis.

The inclusion of any procedure as a covered surgical procedure under §416.65 does not preclude its coverage in an inpatient hospital setting under Medicare.

§416.76 Applicability.

The provisions of this subpart apply to facility services furnished before January 1, 2008.

[71 FR 68226, Nov. 24, 2006]

Subpart E—Prospective Payment System for Facility Services Furnished Before January 1, 2008

§416.120 Basis for payment.

The basis for payment depends on where the services are furnished.

(a) Hospital outpatient department. Payment is in accordance with part 419 of this chapter.

(b) [Reserved]

(c) ASC—(1) General rule. Payment is based on a prospectively determined rate. This rate covers the cost of services such as supplies, nursing services, equipment, etc., as specified in §416.61. The rate does not cover physician services or other medical services covered under part 410 of this chapter (for example, X-ray services or laboratory services) which are not directly related to the performance of the surgical procedures. Those services may be billed separately and paid on a reasonable charge basis.

(2) Single and multiple surgical procedures. (i) If one covered surgical procedure is furnished to a beneficiary in an operative

session, payment is based on the prospectively determined rate for that procedure.

(ii) If more than one surgical procedure is furnished in a single operative session, payment is based on—

(A) The full rate for the procedure with the highest prospectively determined rate; and

(B) One half of the prospectively determined rate for each of the other procedures.

(3) Deductibles and coinsurance. Part B deductible and coinsurance amounts apply as specified in §410.152 (a) and (i) of this chapter.

[56 FR 8844, Mar. 1, 1991; 56 FR 23022, May 20, 1991, as amended at 71 FR 68226, Nov. 24, 2006]

§416.121 Applicability.

The provisions of this subpart apply to facility services furnished before January 1, 2008.

[71 FR 68226, Nov. 24, 2006]

§416.125 ASC facility services payment rate.

(a) The payment rate is based on a prospectively determined standard overhead amount per procedure derived from an estimate of the costs incurred by ambulatory surgical centers generally in providing services furnished in connection with the performance of that procedure.

(b) The payment must be substantially less than would have been paid under the program if the procedure had been performed on an inpatient basis in a hospital.

(c) For services furnished on or after January 1, 2007, and before the effective date of implementation of a revised payment system, the ASC payment rate for a surgical procedure is the lesser of the ASC payment rate established under paragraph (a) of this section or the prospective payment rate for the procedure established under §419.32 of this chapter. The lesser payment amount is determined prior to application of any geographic adjustment.

[56 FR 8844, Mar. 1, 1991, as amended at 71 FR 68226, Nov. 24, 2006]

§416.130 Publication of revised payment methodologies.

Whenever CMS proposes to revise the payment rate for ASCs, CMS publishes a notice in the Federal Register describing the revision. The notice also explains the basis on which the rates were established. After reviewing public comments, CMS publishes a notice establishing the rates authorized by this section. In setting these rates, CMS may adopt reasonable classifications of facilities and may establish different rates for different types of surgical procedures.

[47 FR 34094, Aug. 5, 1982, as amended at 56 FR 8844, Mar. 1, 1991]

§416.140 Surveys.

(a) Timing, purpose, and procedures. (1) No more often than once a year, CMS conducts a survey of a randomly selected sample of participating ASCs to collect data for analysis or reevaluation of payment rates.

(2) CMS notifies the selected ASCs by mail of their selection and of the form and content of the report the ASCs are required to submit within 60 days of the notice.

(3) If the facility does not submit an adequate report in response to CMS's survey request, CMS may terminate the agreement to participate in the Medicare program as an ASC.

(4) CMS may grant a 30-day postponement of the due date for the survey report if it determines that the facility has demonstrated good cause for the delay.

(b) Requirements for ASCs. ASCs must—

(1) Maintain adequate financial records, in the form and containing the data required by CMS, to allow determination of the payment rates for covered surgical procedures furnished to Medicare beneficiaries under this subpart.

(2) Within 60 days of a request from CMS submit, in the form and detail as may be required by CMS, a report of—

(i) Their operations, including the allowable costs actually incurred for the period and the actual number and kinds of surgical procedures furnished during the period; and

(ii) Their customary charges for each surgical procedure furnished for the period.

[47 FR 34094, Aug. 5, 1982, as amended at 56 FR 8845, Mar. 1, 1991]

Subpart F—Coverage, Scope of ASC Services, and Prospective Payment System for ASC Services Furnished on or After January 1, 2008

Source: 72 FR 42545, Aug. 2, 2007, unless otherwise noted.

§416.160 Basis and scope.

(a) Statutory basis. (1) Section 1833(i)(2)(D) of the Act requires the Secretary to implement a revised payment system for payment of surgical services furnished in ASCs. The statute requires that, in the year such system is implemented, the system shall be designed to result in the same amount of aggregate expenditures for such services as would be made if there was no requirement for a revised payment system. The revised payment system shall be implemented no earlier than January 1, 2006, and no later than January 1, 2008. The statute provides that the Secretary may implement a reduction in any annual update for failure to report on quality measures as specified by the Secretary. The statute also requires that, for CY 2011 and each subsequent year, any annual update to the ASC payment system, after application of any reduction in the annual update for failure to report on quality measures as specified by the Secretary, be reduced by a productivity adjustment. There shall be no administrative or judicial review under section 1869 of the Act, section 1878 of the Act, or otherwise of the classification system, the relative weights, payment amounts, and the geographic adjustment factor, if any, of the revised payment system.

(2) Section 1833(a)(1)(G) of the Act provides that, beginning with the implementation date of a revised payment system for ASC facility services furnished in connection with a surgical procedure pursuant to section 1833(i)(1)(A) of the Act, the amount paid shall be 80 percent of the lesser of the actual charge for such services or the amount determined by the Secretary under the revised payment system.

(3) Section 1833(i)(1)(A) of the Act requires the Secretary to specify the surgical procedures that can be performed safely on an ambulatory basis in an ASC.

(4) Section 1834(d) of the Act specifies that, when screening colonoscopies or screening flexible sigmoidoscopies are performed in an ASC or hospital outpatient department, payment shall be based on the lesser of the amount under the fee schedule that would apply to such services if they were performed in a hospital outpatient department in an area or the amount under the fee schedule that would apply to such services if they were performed in an ambulatory surgical center in the same area. Section 1834(d) of the Act also specifies that, in the case of screening flexible sigmoidoscopy and screening colonoscopy services, the payment amounts must not exceed the payment rates established for the related diagnostic services.

(5) Section 1833(a)(1) of the Act requires 100 percent payment for preventive services described in section 1861(ww)(2) of the Act (excluding electrocardiograms) to which the United States Preventive Services Task Force (USPSTF) has given a grade of A or B for any indication or population. Section 1833(b)(1) of the Act also specifies that the Part B deductible shall not apply with respect to preventive services described in section 1861(ww)(2) of the Act (excluding electrocardiograms) to which the USPSTF has given a grade of A or B for any indication or population.

(b) Scope. This subpart sets forth—

(1) The scope of ASC services and the criteria for determining the covered surgical procedures for which Medicare provides payment for the associated facility services and covered ancillary services;

(2) The basis of payment for facility services and for covered ancillary services furnished in an ASC in connection with a covered surgical procedure;

(3) The methodologies by which Medicare determines payment amounts for ASC services.

[72 FR 42545, Aug. 2, 2007, as amended at 75 FR 72264, Nov. 24, 2010; 77 FR 68558, Nov. 15, 2012]

§416.161 Applicability of this subpart.

The provisions of this subpart apply to ASC services furnished on or after January 1, 2008.

§416.163 General rules.

(a) Payment is made under this subpart for ASC services specified in §§416.164(a) and (b) furnished to Medicare beneficiaries by a participating ASC in connection with covered surgical procedures as determined by the Secretary in accordance with §416.166.

(b) Payment for physicians' services and payment for anesthetists' services are made in accordance with part 414 of this subchapter.

(c) Payment for items and services other than physicians' and anesthetists' services, as specified in §416.164(c), is made in accordance with §410.152 of this subchapter.

§416.164 Scope of ASC services.

(a) Included facility services. ASC services for which payment is packaged into the ASC payment for a covered surgical procedure under §416.166 include, but are not limited to—

(1) Nursing, technician, and related services;

(2) Use of the facility where the surgical procedures are performed;

(3) Any laboratory testing performed under a Clinical Laboratory Improvement Amendments of 1988 (CLIA) certificate of waiver;

(4) Drugs and biologicals for which separate payment is not allowed under the hospital outpatient prospective payment system (OPPS);

(5) Medical and surgical supplies not on pass-through status under subpart G of part 419 of this subchapter;

(6) Equipment;

(7) Surgical dressings;

(8) Implanted prosthetic devices, including intraocular lenses (IOLs), and related accessories and supplies not on pass-through status under subpart G of part 419 of this subchapter;

(9) Implanted DME and related accessories and supplies not on pass-through status under subpart G of part 419 of this subchapter;

(10) Splints and casts and related devices;

(11) Radiology services for which separate payment is not allowed under the OPPS and other diagnostic tests or interpretive services that are integral to a surgical procedure, except certain diagnostic tests for which separate payment is allowed under the OPPS;

(12) Administrative, recordkeeping and housekeeping items and services;

(13) Materials, including supplies and equipment for the administration and monitoring of anesthesia; and

(14) Supervision of the services of an anesthetist by the operating surgeon.

(b) Covered ancillary services. Ancillary items and services that are integral to a covered surgical procedure, as defined in §416.166, and for which separate payment is allowed include:

(1) Brachytherapy sources;

(2) Certain implantable items that have pass-through status under the OPPS;

(3) Certain items and services that CMS designates as contractor-priced, including, but not limited to, the procurement of corneal tissue for corneal transplant procedures;

(4) Certain drugs and biologicals for which separate payment is allowed under the OPPS;

(5) Certain radiology services and certain diagnostic tests for which separate payment is allowed under the OPPS.

(c) Excluded services. ASC services do not include items and services outside the scope of ASC services for which payment may be made under part 414 of this subchapter in accordance with §410.152, including, but not limited to—

(1) Physicians' services (including surgical procedures and all preoperative and postoperative services that are performed by a physician);

(2) Anesthetists' services;

(3) Radiology services (other than those integral to performance of a covered surgical procedure);

(4) Diagnostic procedures (other than those directly related to performance of a covered surgical procedure);

(5) Ambulance services;

(6) Leg, arm, back, and neck braces other than those that serve the function of a cast or splint;

(7) Artificial limbs;

(8) Nonimplantable prosthetic devices and DME.

[72 FR 42545, Aug. 2, 2007, as amended at 79 FR 67030, Nov. 10, 2014; 80 FR 70604, Nov. 13, 2015]

§416.166 Covered surgical procedures.

(a) Covered surgical procedures. Effective for services furnished on or after January 1, 2008, covered surgical procedures are those procedures that meet the general standards described in paragraph (b) of this section (whether commonly furnished in an ASC or a physician's office) and are not excluded under paragraph (c) of this section.

(b) General standards. Subject to the exclusions in paragraph (c) of this section, covered surgical procedures are surgical procedures specified by the Secretary and published in the Federal Register and/or via the Internet on the CMS Web site that are separately paid under the OPPS, that would not be expected to pose a significant safety risk to a Medicare beneficiary when performed in an ASC, and for which standard medical practice dictates that the beneficiary would not typically be expected to require active medical monitoring and care at midnight following the procedure.

(c) General exclusions. Notwithstanding paragraph (b) of this section, covered surgical procedures do not include those surgical procedures that—

(1) Generally result in extensive blood loss;

(2) Require major or prolonged invasion of body cavities;

(3) Directly involve major blood vessels;

(4) Are generally emergent or life-threatening in nature;

(5) Commonly require systemic thrombolytic therapy;

(6) Are designated as requiring inpatient care under §419.22(n) of this subchapter;

(7) Can only be reported using a CPT unlisted surgical procedure code; or

(8) Are otherwise excluded under §411.15 of this subchapter.

[72 FR 42545, Aug. 2, 2007, as amended at 76 FR 74582, Nov. 30, 2011]

§416.167   Basis of payment.

(a) Unit of payment. Under the ASC payment system, prospectively determined amounts are paid for ASC services furnished to Medicare beneficiaries in connection with covered surgical procedures. Covered surgical procedures and covered ancillary services are identified by codes established under the Healthcare Common Procedure Coding System (HCPCS). The unadjusted national payment rate is determined according to the methodology described in §416.171. The manner in which the Medicare payment amount and the beneficiary coinsurance amount for each ASC service is determined is described in §416.172.

(b) Ambulatory payment classification (APC) groups and payment weights. (1) ASC covered surgical procedures are classified using the APC groups described in §419.31 of this subchapter.

(2) For purposes of calculating ASC national payment rates under the methodology described in §416.171, except as specified in paragraph (b)(3) of this section, an ASC relative payment weight is determined based on the APC relative payment weight for each covered surgical procedure and covered ancillary service that has an applicable APC relative payment weight described in §419.31 of this subchapter.

(3) Notwithstanding paragraph (b)(2) of this section, the relative payment weights for services paid in accordance with §416.171(d) are determined so that the national ASC payment rate does not exceed the unadjusted nonfacility practice expense amount paid under the Medicare physician fee schedule for such procedures under subpart B of part 414 of this subchapter.

§416.171 Determination of payment rates for ASC services.

(a) Standard methodology. The standard methodology for determining the national unadjusted payment rate for ASC services is to calculate the product of the applicable conversion factor and the relative payment weight established under §416.167(b), unless otherwise indicated in this section.

(1) Conversion factor for CY 2008. CMS calculates a conversion factor so that payment for ASC services furnished in CY 2008 would result in the same aggregate amount of expenditures as would be made if the provisions in this Subpart F did not apply, as estimated by CMS.

(2) Conversion factor for CY 2009 and subsequent calendar years. The conversion factor for a calendar year is equal to the conversion factor calculated for the previous year, updated as follows:

(i) For CY 2009, the update is equal to zero percent.

(ii) For CY 2010 and subsequent calendar years, the update is the Consumer Price Index for All Urban Consumers (U.S. city average) as estimated by the Secretary for the 12-month period ending with the midpoint of the year involved.

(iii) For CY 2014 and subsequent calendar years, the Consumer Price Index for All Urban Consumers update determined under paragraph (a)(2)(ii) of this section is reduced by 2.0 percentage points for an ASC that fails to meet the standards for reporting of ASC quality measures as established by the Secretary for the corresponding calendar year.

(iv) Productivity adjustment. (A) For calendar year 2011 and subsequent years, the Consumer Price Index for All Urban Consumers determined under paragraph (a)(2)(ii) of this section, after application of any reduction under paragraph (a)(2)(iii) of this section, is reduced by the productivity adjustment described in section 1886(b)(3)(B)(xi)(II) of the Act.

(B) The application of the provisions of paragraph (a)(2)(iv)(A) of this section may result in the update being less than zero percent for a year, and may result in payment rates for a year being less than the payment rates for the preceding year.

(b) Exception. The national ASC payment rates for the following items and services are not determined in accordance with paragraph (a) of this section but are paid an amount derived from the payment rate for the equivalent item or service set under the payment system established in part 419 of this subchapter as updated annually in the Federal Register and/or via the Internet on the CMS Web site. If a payment rate is not available, the following items and services are designated as contractor-priced:

(1) Covered ancillary services specified in §416.164(b), with the exception of radiology services and certain diagnostic tests as provided in §416.164(b)(5);

(2) The device portion of device-intensive procedures, which are procedures with a HCPCS code-level device offset of greater than 40 percent when calculated according to the standard OPPS APC rate setting methodology.

(3) Procedures using certain separately paid implantable devices that are approved for transitional pass-through payment in accordance with §419.66 of this subchapter.

(c) Transitional payment rates. (1) ASC payment rates for CY 2008 are a transitional blend of 75 percent of the CY 2007 ASC payment rate for a covered surgical procedure on the CY 2007 ASC list of surgical procedures and 25 percent of the payment rate for the procedure calculated under the methodology described in paragraph (a) of this section.

(2) ASC payment rates for CY 2009 are a transitional blend of 50 percent of the CY 2007 ASC payment rate for a covered surgical procedure on the CY 2007 ASC list of surgical procedures and 50 percent of the payment rate for the procedure calculated under the methodology described in paragraph (a) of this section.

(3) ASC payment rates for CY 2010 are a transitional blend of 25 percent of the CY 2007 ASC payment rate for a covered surgical procedure on the CY 2007 ASC list of surgical procedures and 75 percent of the payment rate for the procedure calculated under the methodology described in paragraph (a) of this section.

(4) The national ASC payment rate for CY 2011 and subsequent calendar years for a covered surgical procedure designated in accordance with §416.166 is the payment rates for the procedure calculated under the methodology described in paragraph (a) of this section.

(5) Covered ancillary services described in §416.164(b) and surgical procedures identified as covered when performed in an ASC under §416.166 for the first time beginning on or after January 1, 2008, are not subject to the transitional payment rates applicable in CYs 2008 through 2010 for ASC facility services.

(d) Limitation on payment rates for office-based surgical procedures and covered ancillary radiology services and certain diagnostic tests. Notwithstanding the provisions of paragraph (a) of this section, for any covered surgical procedure under §416.166 that CMS determines is commonly performed in physicians' offices or for any covered ancillary radiology service or diagnostic test under §416.164(b)(5), excluding those listed in paragraphs (d)(1) and (d)(2) of this section, the national unadjusted ASC payment rates for these procedures and services will be the lesser of the amount determined under paragraph (a) of this section or the amount calculated at the nonfacility practice expense relative value units under §414.22(b)(5)(i)(B) of this chapter multiplied by the conversion factor described in §414.20(a)(3) of this chapter.

(1) The national unadjusted ASC payment rate for covered ancillary radiology services that involve certain nuclear medicine procedures will be the amount determined under paragraph (a) of this section.

(2) The national unadjusted ASC payment rate for covered ancillary radiology services that use contrast agents will be the amount determined under paragraph (a) of this section.

(e) Budget neutrality. (1) For CY 2008, CMS establishes the conversion factor to result in budget neutrality as estimated by CMS in accordance with paragraph (a)(1) of this section.

(2) For CY 2009 and subsequent calendar years, CMS adjusts the ASC relative payment weights under §416.167(b)(2) as needed so that any updates and adjustments made under §419.50(a) of this subchapter are budget neutral as estimated by CMS.

[72 FR 42545, Aug. 2, 2007, as amended at 75 FR 72264, Nov. 24, 2010; 76 FR 74582, Nov. 30, 2011; 77 FR 277, Jan. 4, 2012; 77 FR 68558, Nov. 15, 2012; 79 FR 67030, Nov. 10, 2014; 81 FR 79879, Nov. 14, 2016]

§416.172 Adjustments to national payment rates.

(a) General rule. Contractors adjust the payment rates established for ASC services to determine Medicare program payment and beneficiary coinsurance amounts in accordance with paragraphs (b) through (g) of this section.

(b) Lesser of actual charge or geographically adjusted payment rate. Payments to ASCs equal 80 percent of the lesser of—

(1) The actual charge for the service; or

(2) The geographically adjusted payment rate determined under this subpart.

(c) Geographic adjustment—(1) General rule. Except as provided in paragraph (c)(2) of this section, the national ASC payment rates established under §416.171 for covered surgical procedures are adjusted for variations in ASC labor costs across geographic areas using wage index values, labor and nonlabor percentages, and localities specified by the Secretary.

(2) Exception. The geographic adjustment is not applied to the payment rates set for drugs, biologicals, devices with OPPS transitional pass-through payment status, and brachytherapy sources.

(d) Deductibles and coinsurance. Part B deductible and coinsurance amounts apply as specified in §§410.152(a) and (i)(2) of this subchapter.

(e) Payment reductions for multiple surgical procedures—(1) General rule. Except as provided in paragraph (e)(2) of this section, when more than one covered surgical procedure for which payment is made under the ASC payment system is performed during an operative session, the Medicare program payment amount and the beneficiary coinsurance amount are based on—

(i) 100 percent of the applicable ASC payment amount for the procedure with the highest national unadjusted ASC payment rate; and

(ii) 50 percent of the applicable ASC payment amount for all other covered surgical procedures.

(2) Exception: Procedures not subject to multiple procedure discounting. CMS may apply any policies or procedures used with respect to multiple procedures under the prospective payment system for hospital outpatient department services under Part 419 of this subchapter as may be consistent with the equitable and efficient administration of this part.

(f) Interrupted procedures. (1) Subject to the provisions of paragraph (f)(2) of this section, when a covered surgical procedure or covered ancillary service is terminated prior to completion due to extenuating circumstances or circumstances that threaten the well-being of the patient, the Medicare program payment amount and the beneficiary coinsurance amount are based on one of the following—

(i) The full program and beneficiary coinsurance amounts if the procedure for which anesthesia is planned is discontinued after the induction of anesthesia or after the procedure is started;

(ii) One-half of the full program and beneficiary coinsurance amounts if the procedure for which anesthesia is planned is discontinued after the patient is prepared for surgery and taken to the room where the procedure is to be performed but before the anesthesia is induced; or

(iii) One-half of the full program and beneficiary coinsurance amounts if a covered surgical procedure or covered ancillary service for which anesthesia is not planned is discontinued after the patient is prepared and taken to the room where the service is to be provided.

(2) Beginning CY 2016, if the covered surgical procedure is a device-intensive procedure, the full device portion of the ASC device-intensive procedure is removed prior to determining the Medicare program payment amount and the beneficiary coinsurance amount identified in paragraph (f)(1)(ii) of this section.

(g) Payment adjustment for new technology intraocular lenses (NTIOLs). A payment adjustment will be made for insertion of an IOL approved as belonging to a class of NTIOLs as defined in subpart G.

[72 FR 42545, Aug. 2, 2007, as amended at 80 FR 70604, Nov. 13, 2015]

§416.173   Publication of revised payment methodologies and payment rates.

CMS publishes annually, through notice and comment rulemaking in the Federal Register and/or via the Internet on the CMS Web site, the payment methodologies and payment rates for ASC services and designates the covered surgical procedures and covered ancillary services for which CMS will make an ASC payment and other revisions as appropriate.

[76 FR 74582, Nov. 30, 2011]

§416.178 Limitations on administrative and judicial review.

There is no administrative or judicial review under section 1869 of the Act, section 1878 of the Act, or otherwise of the following:

(a) The classification system;

(b) Relative weights;

(c) Payment amounts; and

(d) Geographic adjustment factors.

§416.179 Payment and coinsurance reduction for devices replaced without cost or when full or partial credit is received.

(a) General rule. CMS reduces the amount of payment for a covered surgical procedure for which CMS determines that a significant portion of the payment is attributable to the cost of an implanted device not on pass-through status under subpart G of part 419 of this subchapter when one of the following situations occur:

(1) The device is replaced without cost to the ASC or the beneficiary;

(2) The ASC receives full credit for the cost of a replaced device; or

(3) The ASC receives partial credit for the cost of a replaced device but only where the amount of the device credit is greater than or equal to 50 percent of the cost of the new replacement device being implanted.

(b) Amount of reduction to the ASC payment for the covered surgical procedure. (1) The amount of the reduction to the ASC payment made under paragraphs (a)(1) and (a)(2) of this section is calculated in the same manner as the device payment reduction that would be applied to the ASC payment for the covered surgical procedure in order to remove predecessor device costs so that the ASC payment amount for a device with pass-through status under §419.66 of this subchapter represents the full cost of the device, and no packaged device payment is provided through the ASC payment for the covered surgical procedure.

(2) The amount of the reduction to the ASC payment made under paragraph (a)(3) of this section is 50 percent of the payment reduction that would be calculated under paragraph (b)(1) of this section.

(c) Amount of beneficiary coinsurance. The beneficiary coinsurance is calculated based on the ASC payment for the covered surgical procedure after application of the reduction under paragraph (b) of this section.

[72 FR 42545, Aug. 2, 2007, as amended at 72 FR 66932, No. 27, 2007]

Subpart G—Adjustment in Payment Amounts for New Technology Intraocular Lenses Furnished by Ambulatory Service Centers

Source: 71 FR 68226, Nov. 24, 2006, unless otherwise noted.

§416.180   Basis and scope.

(a) Basis. This subpart implements section 141 of Public Law 103-432, which provides for adjustments to payment amounts for new technology intraocular lenses (IOLs) furnished at ambulatory surgical centers (ASCs).

(b) Scope. This subpart sets forth—

(1) The process for interested parties to request that CMS review the appropriateness of the ASC facility fee for insertion of an IOL. This process includes a review of whether that payment is reasonable and related to the cost of acquiring a lens determined by CMS as belonging to a class of new technology IOLs;

(2) Factors that CMS considers for determination of a new class of new technology IOLs; and

(3) Application of the payment adjustment.

§416.185   Process for establishing a new class of new technology IOLs.

(a) Announcement of deadline for requests for review. CMS announces the deadline for each year's requests for review of a new class of new technology IOLs in the final rule updating the ASC payment rates for that calendar year.

(b) Announcement of new classes of new technology IOLs for which review requests have been made and solicitation of public comments. CMS announces the requests for review received in a calendar year and the deadline for public comments regarding the requests in the proposed rule updating the ASC payment rates for the following calendar year. The deadline for submission of public comments is 30 days following the date of the publication of the proposed rule.

(c) Announcement of determinations regarding requests for review. CMS announces its determinations for a calendar year in the final rule updating the ASC payment rates for the following calendar year. CMS publishes the codes and effective dates allowed for those lenses recognized by CMS as belonging to a class of new technology IOLs. New classes of new technology IOLs are effective 30 days following the date of publication of the final rule.

§416.190   Request for review of payment amount.

(a) When requests can be submitted. A request for review of the appropriateness of ASC payment for insertion of an IOL that might qualify for a payment adjustment as belonging to a new class of new technology IOLs must be submitted to CMS in accordance with the annual published deadline.

(b) Who may submit a request. Any individual, partnership, corporation, association, society, scientific or academic establishment, or professional or trade organization able to furnish the information required in paragraph (c) of this section may request that CMS review the appropriateness of the payment amount provided under section 1833(i)(2)(A)(iii) of the Act with respect to an IOL that meets the criteria of a new technology IOL under §416.195.

(c) Content of a request. In order to be accepted by CMS for review, a request for review of the ASC payment amount for insertion of an IOL must include all the information as specified by CMS.

(d) Confidential information. In order for CMS to invoke the protection allowed under Exemption 4 of the Freedom of Information Act (5 U.S.C. 552(b)(4)) and, with respect to trade secrets, the Trade Secrets Act (18 U.S.C. 1905), the requestor must clearly identify all information that is to be characterized as confidential.

§416.195 Determination of membership in new classes of new technology IOLs.

(a) Factors to be considered. CMS uses the following criteria to determine whether an IOL qualifies for a payment adjustment as a member of a new class of new technology IOLs when inserted at an ASC:

(1) The IOL is considered new. CMS will evaluate an application for a new technology IOL only if the IOL type has received initial FDA premarket approval within 3 years prior to the new technology IOL application submission date.

(2) The IOL shall have a new lens characteristic in comparison to currently available IOLs. The labeling, which must be approved by FDA, shall contain a claim of a specific clinical benefit imparted by the new lens characteristic.

(3) The IOL is not described by an active or expired class of new technology IOLs; that is, it does not share a predominant, class-defining characteristic associated with improved clinical outcomes with members of an active or expired class.

(4) Any specific clinical benefit referred to in paragraph (a)(2) of this section must be supported by evidence that demonstrates that the IOL results in a measurable, clinically meaningful, improved outcome. Improved outcomes include:

(i) Reduced risk of intraoperative or postoperative complication or trauma;

(ii) Accelerated postoperative recovery;

(iii) Reduced induced astigmatism;

(iv) Improved postoperative visual acuity;

(v) More stable postoperative vision;

(vi) Other comparable clinical advantages.

(b) CMS determination of eligibility for payment adjustment. CMS reviews the information submitted with a completed request for review, public comments submitted timely, and other pertinent information and makes a determination as follows:

(1) The IOL is eligible for a payment adjustment as a member of a new class of new technology IOLs.

(2) The IOL is a member of an active class of new technology IOLs and is eligible for a payment adjustment for the remainder of the period established for that class.

(3) The IOL does not meet the criteria for designation as a new technology IOL and a payment adjustment is not appropriate.

[71 FR 68226, Nov. 24, 2006, as amended at 77 FR 68558, Nov. 15, 2012; 80 FR 70604, Nov. 13, 2015]

§416.200 Payment adjustment.

(a) CMS establishes the amount of the payment adjustment for classes of new technology IOLs through proposed and final rulemaking in connection with ASC facility services.

(b) CMS adjusts the payment for insertion of an IOL approved as belonging to a class of new technology IOLs for the 5-year period of time established for that class.

(c) Upon expiration of the 5-year period of the payment adjustment, payment reverts to the standard rate for IOL insertion procedures performed in ASCs.

(d) ASCs that furnish an IOL designated by CMS as belonging to a class of new technology IOLs must submit claims using billing codes specified by CMS to receive the new technology IOL payment adjustment

Subpart H—Requirements Under the Ambulatory Surgical Center Quality Reporting (ASCQR) Program

Source: 80 FR 70604, Nov. 13, 2015, unless otherwise noted.

§416.300 Basis and scope of subpart.

(a) Statutory basis. Section 1833(i)(2)(D)(iv) and (i)(7) of the Act authorizes the Secretary to implement a revised ASC payment system in a manner so as to provide for a 2.0 percentage point reduction in any annual update for an ASC's failure to report on quality measures in accordance with the Secretary's requirements.

(b) Scope. This subpart contains specific requirements and standards for the ASCQR Program.

§416.305　Participation and withdrawal requirements under the ASCQR Program.

(a) Participation in the ASCQR Program. Except as provided in paragraph (c) of this section, an ambulatory surgical center (ASC) is considered as participating in the ASCQR Program on the ASC submits any quality measure data to the ASCQR Program and has been designated as open in the Certification and Survey Provider Enhanced Reporting system for at least four months prior to the beginning of data collection for a payment determination.

(b) Withdrawal from the ASCQR Program, (1) An ASC may withdraw from the ASCQR Program by submitting to CMS a withdrawal of participation form that can be found in the secure portion of the QualityNet Web site.

(2) An ASC may withdraw from the ASCQR Program any time up to and including August 31 of the year preceding a payment determination.

(3) Except as provided in paragraph (c) of this section, an ASC will incur a 2.0 percentage point reduction in its ASC annual payment update for that payment determination year and any subsequent payment determinations in which it is withdrawn.

(4) An ASC will be considered as rejoining the ASCQR Program if it begins to submit any quality measure data again to the ASCQR Program.

(c) Minimum case volume for program participation. ASCs with fewer than 240 Medicare claims (Medicare primary and secondary payer) per year during an annual reporting period for a payment determination year are not required to participate in the ASCQR

Program for the subsequent annual reporting period for that subsequent payment determination year.

(d) Indian Health Service hospital outpatient department participation. Beginning with the CY 2017 payment determination, Indian Health Service hospital outpatient departments that bill Medicare under the Ambulatory Surgical Center payment system are not considered ASCs for the purposes of the ASCQR Program. These facilities are not required to meet ASCQR Program requirements and will not receive payment reductions under the ASCQR Program.

§416.310 Data collection and submission requirements under the ASCQR Program.

(a) Requirements for claims-based measures using quality data codes (QDCs). (1) ASCs must submit complete data on individual claims-based quality measures through a claims-based reporting mechanism by submitting the appropriate QDCs on the ASC's Medicare claims.

(2) The data collection period for claims-based quality measures reported using QDCs is the calendar year 2 years prior to the payment determination year. Only claims for services furnished in each calendar year paid by the Medicare Administrative Contractor (MAC) by April 30 of the following year of the ending data collection time period will be included in the data used for the payment determination year.

(3) For ASCQR Program purposes, data completeness for claims-based measures using QDCs is determined by comparing the number of Medicare claims (where Medicare is the primary or secondary payer) meeting measure specifications that contain the appropriate QDCs with the number of Medicare claims that meet

measure specifications, but do not have the appropriate QDCs on the submitted Medicare claim. The minimum threshold for successful reporting is that at least 50 percent of Medicare claims meeting measure specifications contain the appropriate QDCs. ASCs that meet this minimum threshold are regarded as having provided complete data for the claims-based measures using QDCs for the ASCQR Program.

(b) Requirements for claims-based measures not using QDCs. The data collection period for claims-based quality measures not using QDCs is paid Medicare fee-for-service claims from the calendar year 2 years prior to the payment determination year. Only claims for services furnished in each calendar year paid by the MAC by April 30 of the following year of the ending data collection time period will be included in the data used for the payment determination.

(c) Requirements for data submitted via an online data submission tool—(1) Requirements for data submitted via a CMS online data submission tool—(i) QualityNet account for Web-based measures. ASCs must maintain a QualityNet account in order to submit quality measure data to the QualityNet Web site for all Web-based measures submitted via a CMS online data submission too. A QualityNet security administrator is necessary to set-up such an account for the purpose of submitting this information.

(ii) Data collection requirements. The data collection time period for quality measures for which data are submitted via a CMS online data submission tool is for services furnished during the calendar year 2 years prior to the payment determination year. Beginning with the CY 2017 payment determination year, data collected must be submitted during the time period of January 1 to May 15 in the year prior to the payment determination year.

(2) Requirements for data submitted via a non-CMS online data submission tool. The data collection time period for ASC-8:

Influenza Vaccination Coverage Among Healthcare Personnel is from October 1 of the year 2 years prior to the payment determination year to March 31 during the year prior to the payment determination year. Data collected must be submitted by May 15 in the year prior to the payment determination year.

(d) Extension or exemption. CMS may grant an extension or exemption for the submission of information in the event of extraordinary circumstances beyond the control of an ASC, or a systematic problem with one of CMS' data collection systems directly or indirectly affects data submission. CMS may grant an extension or exemption as follows:

(1) Upon request of the ASC. ASCs may request an extension or exemption within 90 days of the date that the extraordinary circumstance occurred. Specific requirements for submission of a request for an extension or exemption are available on the QualityNet Web site; or

(2) At the discretion of CMS. CMS may grant extensions or exemptions to ASCs that have not requested them when CMS determines that an extraordinary circumstance has occurred.

(e) Requirements for Outpatient and Ambulatory Surgery Consumer Assessment of Healthcare Providers and Systems (OAS CAHPS) Survey. OAS CAHPS is the Outpatient and Ambulatory Surgical Center Consumer Assessment of Healthcare Providers and Systems survey that measures patient experience of care after a recent surgery or procedure at either a hospital outpatient department or an ambulatory surgical center. Ambulatory surgical centers must use an approved OAS CAHPS survey vendor to administer and submit OAS CAHPS data to CMS.

(1) [Reserved]

(2) CMS approves an application for an entity to administer the OAS CAHPS survey as a vendor on behalf of one or more ambulatory surgical centers when the applicant has met the Minimum Survey Requirements and Rules of Participation that can be found on the official OAS CAHPS Web site, and agrees to comply with the current survey administration protocols that can be found on the official OAS CAHPS Web site. An entity must be approved OAS CAHPS Survey vendor in order to administer the OAS CAHPS Survey and submit data to CMS on behalf of one or more ambulatory surgical centers.

[80 FR 70604, Nov. 13, 2015, as amended at 81 FR 79879, Nov. 14, 2016]

§416.315 Public reporting of data under the ASCQR Program.

Data that an ASC submitted for the ASCQR Program will be made publicly available on a CMS Web site after providing the ASC an opportunity to review the data to be made public. CMS will publicly display ASC data by the National Provider Identifier (NPI) when data are submitted by the NPI. CMS will publicly display ASC data by the CMS Certification Number (CCN) when data are submitted by the CCNs.

§416.320 Retention and removal of quality measures under the ASCQR Program.

(a) General rule for the retention of quality measures. Quality measures adopted for an ASCQR Program measure set for a previous payment determination year are retained in the ASCQR Program for measure sets for subsequent payment determination years, except when they are removed, suspended, or replaced as set forth in paragraphs (b) and (c) of this section.

(b) Immediate measure removal. In cases where CMS believes that the continued use of a measure as specified raises patient safety concerns, CMS will immediately remove a quality measure from the ASCQR Program and will promptly notify ASCs and the public of the removal of the measure and the reasons for its removal through the ASCQR Program ListServ and the ASCQR Program QualityNet Web site. CMS will confirm the removal of the measure for patient safety concerns in the next ASCQR Program rulemaking.

(c) Measure removal, suspension, or replacement through the rulemaking process. Unless a measure raises specific safety concerns as set forth in paragraph (b) of this section, CMS will use the regular rulemaking process to remove, suspend, or replace quality measures in the ASCQR Program to allow for public comment.

(1) Criteria for removal of quality measures. (i) CMS will use the following criteria to determine whether to remove a measure from the ASCQR Program:

(A) Measure performance among ASCs is so high and unvarying that meaningful distinctions and improvements in performance can no longer be made (topped-out measures);

(B) Availability of alternative measures with a stronger relationship to patient outcomes;

(C) A measure does not align with current clinical guidelines or practice;

(D) The availability of a more broadly applicable (across settings, populations, or conditions) measure for the topic;

(E) The availability of a measure that is more proximal in time to desired patient outcomes for the particular topic;

(F) The availability of a measure that is more strongly associated with desired patient outcomes for the particular topic; and

(G) Collection or public reporting of a measure leads to negative unintended consequences other than patient harm.

(ii) The benefits of removing a measure from the ASCQR Program will be assessed on a case-by-case basis. A measure will not be removed solely on the basis of meeting any specific criterion.

(2) Criteria to determine topped-out measures. For the purposes of the ASCQR Program, a measure is considered to be topped-out under paragraph (c)(1)(i)(A) of this section when it meets both of the following criteria:

(i) Statistically indistinguishable performance at the 75th and 90th percentiles (defined as when the difference between the 75th and 90th percentiles for an ASC's measure is within two times the standard error of the full data set); and

(ii) A truncated coefficient of variation less than or equal to 0.10.

§416.325 Measure maintenance under the ASCQR Program.

(a) Measure maintenance under the ASCQR Program. CMS follows different procedures to update the measure specifications under the ASCQR Program based on whether the change is substantive or nonsubstantive. CMS will determine what constitutes a substantive versus a nonsubstantive change to a measure's specifications on a case-by-case basis.

(b) Substantive changes. CMS will continue to use rulemaking to adopt substantive updates to measures in the ASCQR Program.

(c) Nonsubstantive changes. If CMS determines that a change to a measure previously adopted in the ASCQR Program is nonsubstantive, CMS will use a subregulatory process to revise the ASCQR Program Specifications Manual so that it clearly identifies the changes to that measure and provide links to where additional information on the changes can be found. When a measure undergoes subregulatory maintenance, CMS will provide notification of the measure specification update on the QualityNet Web site and in the ASCQR Program Specifications Manual, and will provide sufficient lead time for ASCs to implement the revisions where changes to the data collection systems would be necessary.

§416.330 Reconsiderations under the ASCQR Program.

(a) Reconsiderations of ASCQR Program decisions. An ASC may request reconsideration of a decision by CMS that it has not met the requirements of the ASCQR Program for a particular payment determination year. An ASC must submit a reconsideration request to CMS by no later than the first business day on or after March 17 of the affected payment year.

(b) Requirements for reconsideration requests. A reconsideration request must contain the following information:

(1) The ASC CCN and related NPI(s);

(2) The name of the ASC;

(3) The CMS-identified reason for not meeting the requirements of the ASCQR Program for the affected payment determination year as provided in any CMS notification to the ASC;

(4) The ASC's basis for requesting reconsideration. The ASC must identify its specific reason(s) for believing it met the ASCQR

Program requirements for the affected payment determination year and should not be subject to the reduced ASC annual payment update;

(5) The ASC-designated personnel contact information, including name, email address, telephone number, and mailing address (must include physical mailing address, not just a post office box); and

(6) A copy of all materials that the ASC submitted to comply with the requirements of the affected ASCQR Program payment determination year. With regard to information on claims, ASCs are not required to submit copies of all submitted claims, but instead may focus on the specific claims at issue. For these claims, ASCs should submit relevant information, which could include copies of the actual claims at issue.

(c) Reconsideration process. Upon receipt of a request for reconsideration, CMS will do the following:

(1) Provide an email acknowledgement, using the contact information provided in the reconsideration request, notifying the ASC that the request has been received; and

(2) Provide a formal response to the ASC contact using the information provided in the reconsideration request notifying the ASC of the outcome of the reconsideration process.

(d) Final ASCQR Program payment determination. For an ASC that submits a timely reconsideration request, the reconsideration determination is the final ASCQR Program payment determination. For an ASC that does not submit a timely reconsideration request, the CMS determination is the final payment determination. There is no appeal of any final ASCQR Program payment determination.

Source:

The Conditions for Coverage can be accessed on line at the Electronic Code of Federal Regulations web site for Title 42 – Public Health:

http://www.ecfr.gov/cgi-bin/text-idx?c=ecfr&rgn=div5&view=text&node=42:3.0.1.1.3&idno=42

The regulations related to ambulatory surgery center licensure in Pennsylvania are included in this section.

Authority

The provisions of this Part IV issued under sections 2101—3002 of The Administrative Code of 1929 (71 P. S. §§ 531—732); Articles IX and X of the Public Welfare Code (62 P. S. §§ 901—922 and 1001—1080); and Reorganization Plan No. 3 of 1975, unless otherwise noted.

Source

The provisions of this Part IV adopted August 29, 1975, effective September 1, 1975, 5 Pa.B. 2233, amended February 10, 1977, effective February 12, 1977, 7 Pa.B. 437, unless otherwise noted.

Cross References

This part cited in 28 Pa. Code § 711.2 (relating to policy); 34 Pa. Code § 403.22 (relating to health care facilities); and 55 Pa. Code § 5320.54 (relating to seclusion and restraints).

Subpart A.

GENERAL PROVISIONS

§ 51.1. Legal base, scope and definitions.

(a) This subpart implements the act.

(b) This subpart contains standards which are applicable to all entities licensed as health care facilities under the act. It also identifies specific health care services which are restricted to specified health care facilities.

(c) The following words and terms, when used in this subpart have the following meanings, unless the context clearly indicates otherwise:

Act—The Health Care Facilities Act (35 P. S. §§ 448.101—448.904b).

Department—The Department of Health of the Commonwealth.

§ 51.2. Licensed facilities.

The Department licenses the following health care facilities under the act:

(1)   Ambulatory surgical facilities.

(2)   General hospitals.

(3)   Special hospitals.

(4)   Long-term care nursing facilities.

(5)   Birth centers.

(6)   Home health care agencies.

(7)   Cancer treatment centers.

§ 51.3. Notification.

(a) A health care facility shall notify the Department in writing at least 60 days prior to the intended commencement of a health care service which has not been previously provided at that facility.

(b) A health care facility shall notify the Department in writing at least 60 days prior to the intended date of providing services in new beds it intends to add to its approved complement of beds.

(c) A health care facility shall provide similar notice at least 60 days prior to the effective date it intends to cease providing an existing health care service or reduce its licensed bed complement.

(d) A health care facility shall submit to the Department architectural plans and blueprints of proposed new construction, alteration or renovation to the facility. This material shall be submitted at least 60 days before the initiation of construction, alteration or renovation. The Department will review these documents to assure compliance with relevant life safety code and other regulatory requirements. The Department will respond to the facility by either issuing an approval or disapproval or requesting further information within 45 days of receipt of the facility's submission. The facility may not initiate construction, alteration or renovation until it has received an approval from the Department.

(e) If a health care facility is aware of information which shows that the facility is not in compliance with any of the Department's regulations which are applicable to that health care facility, and that the noncompliance seriously com- promises quality assurance or patient safety, it shall immediately notify the Department in writing of its noncompliance. The notification shall include sufficient detail and information to alert the Department as to the reason for the failure to comply and the steps which the health care facility shall take to bring it into compliance with the regulation.

(Editor's Note: Under section 314 of the act of March 20, 2002 (P. L. 154, No.13) (act), subsections (f) and (g) are abrogated with respect to a medical facility upon the reporting of a serious event, incident or infrastructure failure pursuant to section 313 of the act.)

(f) If a health care facility is aware of a situation or the occurrence of an event at the facility which could seriously compromise quality assurance or patient safety, the facility shall immediately notify the Department in writing. The notification shall include sufficient detail and information to alert the Department as to the reason for its occurrence and the steps which the health care facility shall take to rectify the situation.

(g) For purposes of subsections (e) and (f), events which seriously compromise quality assurance or patient safety include, but are not limited to, the following:

(1)   Deaths due to injuries, suicide or unusual circumstances.

(2)   Deaths due to malnutrition, dehydration or sepsis.

(3)   Deaths or serious injuries due to a medication error.

(4)   Elopements.

(5)   Transfers to a hospital as a result of injuries or accidents.

(6)   Complaints of patient abuse, whether or not confirmed by the facility.

(7)   Rape.

(8)   Surgery performed on the wrong patient or on the wrong body part. (9) Hemolytic transfusion reaction.

(10) Infant abduction or infant discharged to the wrong family.

(11) Significant disruption of services due to disaster such as fire,

storm, flood or other occurrence.

(12) Notification of termination of any services vital to the continued safe operation of the facility or the health and safety of its patients and personnel, including, but not limited to, the anticipated or actual termination of electric, gas, steam heat, water, sewer and local exchange telephone service.

(13) Unlicensed practice of a regulated profession.

(14) Receipt of a strike notice.

(h) A health care facility shall send the written notification required under subsections (a)—(f) to the director of the division in the Department responsible for the licensure of the health care facility.

(i) Information contained in the notification submitted to the Department by a facility under subsection (e) or (f) may not, unless otherwise ordered by a court for good cause shown, be produced for inspection or copying by, nor may the contents thereof be disclosed to, a person other than the Secretary, the Secretary's representative or another government agency, without the consent of the facility which filed the report.

(j) The Secretary and the Secretary's representative shall use the information contained in the notification from the facility only in connection with the enforcement of the Department's responsibilities under the act, or other applicable statutes within the Department's jurisdiction.

(k) The notification requirements of this section do not require a facility, in providing a notification under subsection (e) or (f), to include information which is deemed confidential and not reportable to the Department under other provisions of Federal or

State law or regulations.

(l) A health care facility may not commence the provision of new health care services or provide services in new beds until it has been informed by the Department that it is in compliance with all licensure requirements.

Cross References

This section cited in 28 Pa. Code § 201.14 (relating to responsibility of licensee).

§ 51.4. Change in ownership; change in management.

(a) A health care facility shall notify the Department in writing at least 30 days prior to transfer involving 5% or more of the stock or equity of the health care facility.

 (b) A health care facility shall notify the Department in writing at least 30 days prior to a change in ownership or a change in the form of ownership or name of the facility. A change in ownership shall mean any transfer of the con- trolling interest in a health care facility.

(c) A health care facility shall notify the Department in writing within 30 days after a change of management of a health care facility. A change in management occurs when the person responsible for the day to day operation of the health care facility changes.

§ 51.5. Building occupancy.

(a) New construction, alterations or renovations that provide space for patient or resident rooms or services may not be used or occupied until authorization for the occupancy has been received from the Department.

(b) A health care facility shall request a preoccupancy survey at least 30 days prior to the anticipated occupancy of the facility or an addition or remodeled part thereof. The Department will conduct an onsite survey of the new or remodeled portion of the health care facility prior to granting approval for occupancy. The Department may give the authorization to occupy the new or remodeled portion of the health care facility by an interim written authorization. If interim authorization for occupancy is given, the Department will provide the health care facility with formal authorization within 30 days.

Cross References

This section cited in 28 Pa. Code § 571.11 (relating to principle); and 34 Pa. Code § 403.22 (relating to health care facilities).

§ 51.6. Identification of personnel.

(a) When working in a health care facility and when clinically feasible, the following individuals shall wear an identification tag which displays that person's name and professional designation:

(1) Health care practitioners licensed or certified by Commonwealth agencies.

(2) Health care providers employed by health care facilities.

(b) The identification tag shall include the individual's full name. Abbreviated professional designations may be used only when the designation indicates licensure or certification by a Commonwealth agency, otherwise the full title shall be printed on the tag.

(c) The last name of the individual may be omitted or concealed when treating patients who exhibit symptoms of irrationality or violence.

Cross References

This section cited in 28 Pa. Code § 53.2 (relating to requirements).(359597) No. 447 Feb. 12

CIVIL RIGHTS

§ 51.11. Civil rights compliance.

A health care facility shall comply with all civil rights laws. The Department may make onsite visits at its discretion to verify the civil rights compliance status of the health care facility.

§ 51.12. Nondiscriminatory policy.

(a) A health care facility shall have a nondiscriminatory policy which applies to all patients or residents and staff. The policy shall include a prohibition on the segregation of buildings, wings, floors and rooms for reasons of race, color, national origin, ancestry, age, sex, religion, handicap or disability. The nondiscriminatory policy shall also address the following:

(1) Inpatient or outpatient admission or care.

(2) Assigning patients or residents to rooms, floors and sections.

(3) Asking patients or residents about roommate preferences.

(4) Assignments of staff to patient or resident services.

(5)   Staff privileges of professionally qualified personnel.

(6)   Utilization of the health care facility.

(7)   Transfers of patients or residents from their rooms.

(b) A health care facility is required to comply with Title VI of the Civil Rights Act of 1964 (42 U.S.C.A. §§ 2000e—2000e-17) and the Pennsylvania Human Relations Act (43 P. S. §§ 951—962.2) and to sign the following statement prior to receiving an initial license:

"This facility has agreed to comply with the provisions of the Federal Civil Rights Act of 1964 and the Pennsylvania Human Relations Act and all requirements imposed pursuant thereto to the end that no person shall, on the grounds of race, color, national origin, ancestry, age, sex, religious creed, or disability, be excluded from participation in, be denied benefits of, or otherwise be subject to discrimination in the provision of any care or service."

Cross References

This section cited in 28 Pa. Code § 51.13 (relating to civil rights compliance records).

§ 51.13. Civil rights compliance records.

(a) A health care facility shall maintain the following records to show compliance with § 51.12 (relating to nondiscriminatory policy):

(1) A copy of the health care facility's admission policy which includes the date of its adoption, which sets forth in clear terms nondiscriminatory practices with regard to race, color, national origin, creed, ancestry, age, sex, religion, handicap or disability.

(2) A copy of a signed and dated notification to employees of the health care facility's nondiscrimination policy.

(3) Evidence that the nondiscriminatory practices of the health care facility have been publicized in the community at least every 3 years by one of the following methods: newspapers, television, radio, brochure or yellow pages.

(b) Copies of the health care facility's nondiscriminatory policy shall be posted in locations accessible to the facility's staff and the general public.

(c) The health care facility shall provide the Department with a signed and dated copy of the nondiscriminatory policy within 30 days of the effective date of any change in the policy.

RESTRICTION OF PROVISION OF HEALTH CARE SERVICES

§ 51.21. Surgery.

Surgery shall be performed only in an acute care hospital or in a Class A, Class B or Class C ambulatory surgical facility.

§ 51.22. Cardiac catheterization.

Cardiac catheterization shall be performed only in an acute care hospital.

§ 51.23. Positron emission tomography.

Positron emission tomography (PET) scanning services shall be provided only in a hospital which complies with the regulations of the Department governing radiology and nuclear medicine services.

§ 51.24. Lithotripsy.

Lithotripsy services shall be provided only in a hospital or ambulatory surgical facility authorized to provide anesthesia services under its license.

§ 51.31. Principle.

EXCEPTIONS

The Department may grant exceptions to this part when the policy and objectives contained therein are otherwise met, or when compliance would create an unreasonable hardship and an exception would not impair or endanger the health, safety or welfare of a patient or resident. No exceptions or departures from this part will be granted if compliance with the requirement is provided for by statute.

Cross References

This section cited in 28 Pa. Code § 136.11 (relating to director); 28 Pa. Code § 138.11 (relating to director); 28 Pa. Code § 139.3 (relating to director); and 28 Pa. Code § 158.11 (relating to medical director).

§ 51.32. Exceptions for innovative programs.

This part is not intended to restrict the efforts of a health care facility to develop innovative and improved programs of management, clinical practice, physical renovation or structural design. Whenever this part appears to preclude a program which may improve the capacity of the health care facility to deliver higher quality care and services or to operate more efficiently without compromising patient or resident care, the Department encourages the health care facility to request appropriate exceptions under this chapter.

Notes of Decisions

Generally

Multiple hospitals filed petition for review in the nature of an action for mandamus against the

Department of Health and others to require the Department to comply with provision in the 2005

General Appropriation Bill compelling Department and others to use portion of appropriations for the

"negotiation of criteria under the angioplasty demonstration project"; however, because bill sought to compel Department to undertake actions in particular way, the appropriation conflicted with the Health Care Facilities Act that gave Department exclusive jurisdiction over health care providers and was, therefore, unconstitutional. Uniontown Hospital v. Department of Health, 905 A.2d 560, 565 (Pa. Cmwlth. 2006).

Cross References

This section cited in 28 Pa. Code § 51.13 (relating to civil rights compliance records); 28 Pa. Code

§ 136.11 (relating to director); 28 Pa. Code § 138.11 (relating to director); 28 Pa. Code § 139.3 (relating to director); and 28 Pa. Code § 158.11 (relating to medical director).

§ 51.33. Requests for exceptions.

(a) A health care facility shall make requests for exceptions to the Department in writing.

(b) The Department will retain the requests on file and document whether they have been approved or disapproved.

(c) Upon receipt of a request for exceptions, the request will be published in the Pennsylvania Bulletin with a public comment period. The Department will review these comments before making a determination to approve or disapprove an exception. The Department will publish requests for exceptions in emergency situations, but will not include a public comment period.

(d) The Department will publish notice of all approved exceptions in the Pennsylvania Bulletin on a periodic basis.

(e) The health care facility shall retain approved requests on file during the period the exception remains in effect.

Cross References

This section cited in 28 Pa. Code § 136.11 (relating to director); 28 Pa. Code § 138.11 (relating to director); 28 Pa. Code § 139.3 (relating to director); and 28 Pa. Code § 158.11 (relating to medical director).

§ 51.34. Revocation of exceptions.

(a) An exception granted under this chapter may be revoked by the Department for justifiable reason. The Department will provide notice of the revocation in writing and will include the reason for the revocation and the date upon which the exception will be terminated.

(b) In revoking an exception, the Department will provide for a reasonable period of time between the date of written notice of the revocation and the date of termination of an exception to afford the health care facility an opportunity to come into compliance with the applicable regulations.

(c) If a health care facility wishes to request a reconsideration of a denial or revocation of an exception, it shall do so in writing to the director of the appropriate division within 30 days after service of the adverse notification.

Cross References

This section cited in 28 Pa. Code § 136.11 (relating to director); 28 Pa. Code § 138.11 (relating to director); 28 Pa. Code § 139.3 (relating to director); and 28 Pa. Code § 158.11 (relating to medical director).

§ 51.41. Violations, penalties.

SANCTIONS

(a) When appropriate, the Department will work with the health care facility to rectify a violation of this part.

(b) A health care facility that violates this part may be subject to sanctions by the Department, which include:

(1) Suspension of its license.

(2) Revocation of its license.

(3) Refusal to renew its license.

(4) Limitation of its license as to operation of a portion of the health care facility or to the services which may be provided at the health care facility.

(5) Issuance of a provisional license.

(6) Submission of a plan of correction.

(7) Limitation or suspension of admissions to the health care facility.

(c) A person who violates this part may be subject to a civil penalty, not to exceed $500 per day.

CHAPTER 53.

PHOTO IDENTIFICATION BADGES

Authority

This chapter 53 issued under sections 803(2) and 809.2 of the Health Care Facilities Act (35 P. S. §§ 448.803(2) and 448.809b), unless otherwise noted.

Source

This chapter 53 adopted December 9, 2011, effective December 10, 2011, 41 Pa.B. 6672, unless otherwise noted.

§ 53.1. Legal basis, scope and definitions.

(a) This chapter implements section 809.2 of the act (35 P. S. § 448.809b). (b) This chapter contains standards which are applicable to the following:

(1) All entities licensed as health care facilities under the act.

(2) The private practice of a physician.

(c) The following words and terms, when used in this chapter, have the following meanings:

Direct care—The actual delivery of health care services or assistance with activities of daily living to a consumer or patient.

Employee—An employee or a physician of any of the following who delivers direct care to a consumer:

(i) A health care facility.

(ii) A health care provider.

(iii) The private practice of a physician. (iv) An employment agency.

Employment agency—A public or private organization that provides employment services for persons seeking employment and for potential employers seeking employees who provide direct care to consumers.

Employment status—Full-time, part-time, temporary, contractual or other classification of work that indicates the relationship between the employee and the health care facility, health care provider or employment agency.

Health care facility—A facility licensed by the Department under the act.

Health care provider—An individual, a trust or estate, a partnership, a corporation (including associations, joint stock companies and insurance companies), the Commonwealth or a political subdivision or instrumentality (including a municipal corporation or authority) thereof, that operates a health care facility.

Outside of the health care facility or employment agency—Health care services that are provided to patients and consumers at a location other than a health care facility or employment agency, such as at the patient or consumer's residence.

Private practice of a physician—

(i) A circumstance in which a health care practitioner or an employee under a health care practitioner's supervision provides direct care to a patient or consumer.

(ii) This does not include a physician practice group which is owned and operated by a health care provider.

Title—A license, certification or registration held by the employee.

§ 53.2. Requirements.

(a) This chapter applies to an employee who delivers direct care as follows:

(1) Outside of a health care facility or employment agency.

(2) In a health care facility.

(3) At the private practice of a physician.

(b) An employee who delivers direct care outside of a health care facility or employment agency or at the private practice of a physician shall wear a photo identification badge that meets the requirements in § 53.3 (relating to contents of photo identification badge).

(c) An employee who delivers direct care in a health care facility shall wear an identification badge that meets the requirements in § 51.6 (relating to identification of personnel).

§ 53.3. Contents of photo identification badge.

(a) An employee's photo identification badge must include the following:

(1) A recent photograph of the employee, updated as provided for in sub- section (c).

(2) The employee's full name to include, at a minimum, the full first and last name.

(3) The employee's title.

(4) The name of the employee's health care facility or employment agency. (b) The identification badge issued by an employment agency for an employee who is providing direct care for a health care facility must include the items in subsection (a). In addition, the health care facility where the employee of the employment agency is working shall issue the employee an identification badge that contains the name of the health care facility, the employment status of the employee at that facility and the employee's title.

(c) Photographs shall be updated at least every 4 years.

Cross References

This section cited in 28 Pa. Code § 53.2 (relating to requirements); and 28 Pa. Code § 53.5 (relating to exceptions).

§ 53.4. (Reserved).

§ 53.5. Exceptions.

(a) Photograph. A health care facility, health care provider, employment agency or private practice of a physician may permit an employee to wear an identification badge without a photograph if having a photograph taken would violate the tenets of the employee's religion or religious beliefs.

(b) Policies and procedures for exemption. A health care facility, health care provider, employment agency or private practice of a physician shall establish policies and procedures in the event that an employee requests an exception under subsection (a), which, at a minimum:

(1) Require the employee to submit a signed and notarized statement that the taking of a photograph would violate the employee's religion or religious beliefs.

(2) Ensure that the employee wears an identification badge that contains the information in § 53.3(a)(2)−(4) (relating to contents of photo identification badge).

(3) Contain the employee's height and eye color.

(c) Use of identification badge not clinically feasible. An employee may not be required to wear an identification badge while delivering direct care to a patient or consumer if not clinically feasible.

(d) Employee safety. The last name of the employee may be omitted or concealed when delivering direct care to a patient or consumer who exhibits symptoms of irrationality or violence.

(e) Policies and procedures for exemption. A health care facility, health care provider, employment agency or private practice of a physician shall establish policies and procedures in the event that an employee requires an exception under subsection (d), which, at a minimum describe:

(1) The process to be followed in the event that an employee

requires an exception.

(2) How employees with the same first name will be differentiated.

Subpart F.

AMBULATORY SURGICAL FACILITIES

Authority

The provisions of this Subpart F issued under Chapter 8 of the Health Care Facilities Act (35 P. S. §§ 448.801a—448.820), specifically sections 448.801a and 448.803; and section 2102(a) and (g) of The Administrative Code of 1929 (71 P. S. § 532(a) and (g)), unless otherwise noted.

Source

The provisions of this Subpart F adopted January 23, 1987, effective March 25, 1987, 17 Pa.B. 376, unless otherwise noted.

CHAPTER 551.

GENERAL INFORMATION GENERAL PROVISIONS

Source

The provisions of this Chapter 551 adopted January 23, 1987, effective March 25, 1987, 17 Pa.B. 376, unless otherwise noted.

GENERAL PROVISIONS

§ 551.1. Legal base.

(a) This subpart is promulgated by the Department under Chapter 8 of the act (35 P. S. §§ 448.801—448.820), and section 2102(a) and (g) of The Administrative Code of 1929 (71 P. S. § 532(a) and (g)).

(b) The Department has the duty to promulgate regulations necessary to implement Chapter 8 of the act and to assure that its regulations and the act are enforced.

(c) The purpose of this subpart is to protect and promote the public health and welfare through the establishment and enforcement of regulations setting minimum standards in the construction, maintenance and operation of ASFs. The standards are intended to assure safe, adequate and efficient facilities and services, and to promote the health, safety and adequate care of the patients of the facilities. It is also the purpose of this subpart to assure quality health care through appropriate and nonduplicative review and inspection, with regard to the protection of the health and rights of privacy of the patients and without unreasonably interfering with the operation of the ambulatory surgical facility.

Source

The provisions of this § 551.1 amended October 22, 1999, effective November 22, 1999, 29 Pa.B. 5583. Immediately preceding text appears at serial pages (251633) to (251634).

§ 551.2. Affected institutions.

(a) This subpart applies to ASFs, profit or nonprofit, operated within this Commonwealth. Only those facilities which are licensed under this subpart shall provide ambulatory surgery in this Commonwealth, except as provided in Class A facilities.

(b) This subpart does not apply to outpatient surgery performed at licensed hospitals, or to dentists' or oral surgeons' offices except to the extent the offices seek licensure as ASFs.

Source

The provisions of this § 551.2 amended October 22, 1999, effective November 22, 1999, 29 Pa.B.5583. Immediately preceding text appears at serial page (251634).

§ 551.3. Definitions.

The following words and terms, when used in this subpart, have the following meanings, unless the context clearly indicates otherwise:

ASF—Ambulatory surgical facility—

(i)   A facility or portion thereof not located upon the premises of a hospital which provides specialty or multispecialty outpatient surgical treatment. (ii)This does not include individual or group practice offices of private physicians or dentists, unless the offices have a distinct part used solely for outpatient surgical treatment on a regular and organized basis. For the purposes of this provision, outpatient surgical treatment means treatment to patients who do not require hospitalization, but who require constant medical supervision following the surgical procedure performed.

Act—The Health Care Facilities Act (35 P. S. §§ 448.101—448.904).

Ambulatory surgery—Surgery which is performed:

(i) On an outpatient basis in a facility which is not located in a hospital.

(ii) On patients who do not require hospitalization but who do require constant medical supervision following the surgical

procedure performed and whose total length of stay does not exceed the standards in this subpart. Anesthesia—The use of pharmaceutical agents to induce the loss of sensation. For the purpose of this chapter, the term applies when any patient, in any setting receives, for any purpose, by any route, one of the following:
(i)   General, spinal or other regional anesthesia.

(ii) Sedation (with or without analgesia), for which there is a reasonable expectation that, in the manner used, will result in the loss of protective reflexes for a significant percentage of a group of patients.

Anesthesiologist—A physician licensed by the State Board of Medicine under the Medical Practice Act of 1985 (63 P. S. §§ 422.1—422.45) who has completed an accredited residency training program in anesthesia.

Anesthetist—A generic term used to identify anesthesiologists, nurse anesthetists or dentist anesthetists.

Authenticate—To verify authorship for example by written signature, identifiable initials or computer key.

Authorized person to administer drugs and medications—In an ASF, the term includes the following:

(i) Persons who are currently licensed or certified by the Bureau of Professional and Occupational Affairs, Department of State, and whose scope of practice includes the administration of drugs.

(ii) Registered nurses who are currently licensed by the Bureau of Professional and Occupational Affairs, Department of State.

(iii) Practical nurses who have successfully passed the State Board of Nursing examination.

(iv) Practical nurses licensed by waiver in this Commonwealth who have successfully passed the United States Public Health Service Proficiency Examination.

(v) Practical nurses licensed by waiver in this Commonwealth who have successfully passed a medication course approved by the State Board of Nursing.

(vi) Student nurses of approved nursing programs who are functioning under the direct supervision of a member of the school faculty who is present in the facility.

(vii) Recent graduates of approved nursing programs who are functioning under the direct supervision of a professional nurse who is present in the facility and who possesses valid temporary practice permits. The permits shall expire if the holders of the permits fail the licensing examinations.

(viii) Physician assistants and registered nurse practitioners who are certified by the Bureau of Professional and Occupational Affairs.

Board certified—A physician licensed to practice medicine or osteopathic medicine in this Commonwealth who has successfully passed an examination and has maintained certification in the relevant specialty or subspecialty area, or both, recognized by one of the following groups:

(i) The American Board of Medical Specialties. (ii) The American Osteopathic Association.

(iii) The foreign equivalent of either group listed in subparagraph (i) or (ii).

Classification levels—ASFs shall be classified as follows:

(i) Class A—A private or group practice office of practitioners where procedures performed are limited to those requiring administration of either local or topical anesthesia, or no anesthesia at all and during which reflexes are not obtunded.

(ii) Class B—A single-specialty or multiple-specialty facility with a distinct part used solely for ambulatory surgical treatments involving administration of sedation analgesia or dissociative drugs wherein reflexes may be obtunded; and where patients are limited to Physical Status (PS) PS-I or PS-II patients, unless the patient's PS status would not be adversely affected or sought to be remedied by the surgery. A Class B ASF may be a distinct part of a private or group practice medical or dental office so long as the requirements of this subpart are met.

(iii) Class C—A single-specialty or multiple-specialty facility used exclusively for the purpose of providing ambulatory surgical treatments which involve the use of a spectrum of anesthetic agents, up to and including general anesthesia and where patients are limited to physical status (PS) PS-1, PS-2 or PS-3 patients.

Classification system—A process used to identify three levels of ASFs (A, B and C) based on the procedure, patient status and anesthesia used.

Clinical privileges—Permission to independently render medical care in the ASF which is granted by the governing body under § 553.4(c) and (d) (relating to other functions).

Compliance directive—A directive issued by the Department, citing deficiencies which have come to the attention of the Department through the survey process, or by onsite inspection and directing the ASF to take corrective action as the Department directs or to submit a plan of correction.

Deficiency—A condition which exists contrary to, in violation of, or in non- compliance with this subpart.

Dentist—A person licensed by the State Board of Dentistry under The Dental Law (63 P. S. §§ 120—130b).

Dentist anesthetist—A person licensed by the State Board of Dentistry who has met the requirements for providing anesthesia care services in accordance with the regulations of that Board.

Department—The Department of Health of the Commonwealth.

Distinct part—An area which is part of a practitioner's office which is physically identifiable and where surgery is performed on a regular and organized basis.

Drug administration—An act in which a single dose of an identified drug is given to a patient.

Drug dispensing—The issuance of one or more doses of a prescribed medication under §§ 25.41—25.101.

Facilities—Buildings, equipment and supplies necessary for implementation of ASF services.

Governing body—The individuals, group or entity that has ultimate authority and responsibility for establishing policy, maintaining quality patient care and providing for organizational management and planning.

Graduate nurse—A graduate of an approved program of

professional nursing practicing the profession under The Professional Nursing Law (63 P. S. §§ 221–225).

Licensed practical nurse—A person licensed to practice practical nursing under The Practical Nurse Law (63 P. S. §§ 651–667).

Medical—Pertaining to the practice of medicine, osteopathy, podiatry or dentistry.

Medical staff—The organized group of practitioners who has been appointed by the governing body of the ASF to function under §§ 555.1–555.3 (relating to principle; medical staff membership; and requirements for membership and privileges).

NFPA—The National Fire Protection Association.

New construction—New buildings, additions to existing buildings, conversion of existing buildings or portions thereof or portions of buildings undergoing alterations other than repair.

Nurse anesthetist—A registered nurse licensed by the State Board of Nursing providing anesthesia care in accordance with the requirements of the regulations of that Board.

Nurse practitioner—A person who has been certified by the State Board of Nursing and the State Board of Medicine to perform acts of medical diagnosis or prescription of medical, therapeutic or corrective measure in collaboration with and under the direction of a physician licensed to practice medicine in this Commonwealth, under the Medical Practice Act of 1985 and The Professional Nursing Law.

Nursing services—Patient care aspects of nursing that are performed by registered nurses or by licensed practical nurses and ancillary nursing personnel under the direct supervision of a registered nurse.

Organized—Administratively and functionally structured to include the following:

(i)   Governing body.

(ii) Medical staff.

(iii) Quality assurance.

(iv) Nursing services.

(v)   Pharmacy services.

(vi) Medical record services.

(vii) Laboratory and radiology services.

(viii) Environmental services.

(ix) Fire and safety services.

Outpatient surgical treatment—Surgical procedures performed upon patients who do not require hospitalization but who require constant medical supervision following the surgical procedure performed.

Person in charge—The individual appointed by the governing body to act in its behalf in the overall management of the ASF.

Pharmacist—A person licensed to engage in the practice of pharmacy in this

Commonwealth under The Pharmacy Act (63 P. S. §§ 390.1—390.13).

Pharmacy—A place where the practice of pharmacy is conducted under The Pharmacy Act.

Physical status classifications—The evaluation of the patient's overall health as it would influence the conduct and outcome of anesthesia or surgery, or both. Physical status shall be defined within one of five assigned classes which are:

(i) Class 1 patients have no organic, physiologic, biochemical, metabolic or psychiatric disturbance. The operation to be performed is for a local pathologic process and has no systemic effect.

(ii) Class 2 patients have a systemic disturbance which may be of a mild to moderate degree but which is either controlled or has not changed in its severity for some time.

(iii) Class 3 patients suffer from significant systemic disturbance, although the degree to which it limits the patient's functioning or causes dis- ability may not be quantifiable.

(iv) Class 4 patients suffer from severe systemic diseases that are already life-threatening and may or may not be correctable by surgery.

(v) Class 5 patients are moribund and not expected to survive without surgery.

Physician—A doctor of medicine or osteopathy who holds a current and valid license to practice in this Commonwealth.

Physician assistant—A person who has been certified by the State Board of Medicine or the State Board of Osteopathic Medical Examiners to assist a physician or group of physicians under The

Medical Practice Act of 1985 or The Osteopathic Medical Practice Act (63 P. S. §§ 271.1—271.18).

Podiatrist—A person licensed by the State Board of Podiatry Examiners to practice podiatry under The Podiatry Act of 1956 (63 P. S. §§ 42.1—42.21a).

Practitioner—A licensed physician, dentist or podiatrist.

Preboard certification status—A physician licensed to practice medicine or osteopathic medicine in this Commonwealth who has completed the requirements necessary to take a certification examination offered by a specialty board recognized by the American Board of Medical Specialties, the American Osteopathic Association or the foreign equivalent of either group, and who has been eligible to take the examination for no longer than 3 years.

Premises of a hospital—Buildings, equipment and supplies licensed as a hospital to provide inpatient and outpatient services.

Professional nurse/registered nurse—A person licensed to practice professional nursing under The Professional Nursing Law.

Provider—An individual; a trust or estate; a partnership; a corporation including associations, joint stock companies, health maintenance organizations, professional health service plan corporations and insurance companies; the Commonwealth or a political subdivision or instrumentality thereof, including a municipal corporation or authority that operates an ambulatory surgical facility; and any other legal entity that operates an ambulatory surgical facility.

Secretary—The Secretary of the Department.

Surgery—The branch of medicine that diagnoses and treats

diseases, disorders, malformations and injuries wholly or partially by operative procedures.

Survey—The process of evaluation or reevaluation of the compliance of an ASF with this subpart.

Source

The provisions of this § 551.3 amended October 22, 1999, effective November 22, 1999, 29 Pa.B. 5583. Immediately preceding text appears at serial pages (251634) to (251637).

Cross References

This section cited in 28 Pa. Code § 555.32 (relating to administration of anesthesia).

§§ 551.11—551.13. [Reserved].

Source

The provisions of these §§ 551.11—551.13 reserved October 22, 1999, effective November 22, 1999, 29 Pa.B. 5583. Immediately preceding text appears at serial page (251637).

INTERPRETATIONS

§ 551.21. Criteria for ambulatory surgery.

(a) Ambulatory surgical procedures are limited to those that do not exceed:

(1)   A total of 4 hours of operating time.

(2)   A total of 4 hours directly supervised recovery.

(b) The time limits in subsection (a) may be exceeded only if the patient's condition demands care or recovery beyond the 4-hour limit and the need for the additional time could not have been anticipated prior to surgery.

(c) If the surgical procedures require anesthesia, the anesthesia shall be one of the following:

(1) Local or regional anesthesia.

(2) General anesthesia of 4 hours or less duration.

(d) Surgical procedures may not be of a type that:

(1) Are associated with the risk of extensive blood loss.

(2) Require major or prolonged invasion of body cavities.

(3) Directly involve major blood vessels.

(4) Are emergency or life threatening in nature, unless no hospital is avail- able for the procedure and the need for the surgery could not have been anticipated.

(e) In obtaining informed consent, the practitioner performing the surgery is responsible for disclosure of:

(1) The risks, benefits and alternatives associated with the anesthesia which will be administered.

(2) The risks, benefits and alternatives associated with the procedure which will be performed.

(3) The comparative risks, benefits and alternatives associated with per- forming the procedure in the ASF instead of in a hospital.

(f) The Department may issue interpretations of this subpart, which apply to the question of whether the performance of certain surgical procedures will require licensure as an ASF.

(g) Interpretations issued under this section do not constitute an exercise of delegated legislative power by the Department and will expressly be subject to modification by the Department in an adjudicative proceeding based upon the particular facts and circumstances relevant to a proceeding. Interpretations are not intended to be legally enforceable against a person by the Department. In issuing an adjudication, the Department may consider, but is not bound by, interpretations.

(h) Interpretations adopted by the Department under this section will be reviewed for form and legality under the Commonwealth Attorneys Act (71 P. S.

§§ 732.101—732-506) and, upon approval, will be submitted to the Legislative Reference Bureau for recommended publication in the Pennsylvania Bulletin and Pennsylvania Code as a statement of policy of the Department as a part of this subpart.

Source

The provisions of this § 551.21 amended October 22, 1999, effective November 22, 1999, 29 Pa.B. 5583. Immediately preceding text appears at serial page (251638).

Cross References

This section cited in 28 Pa. Code § 551.22 (relating to criteria for performance of ambulatory surgery on pediatric patients).

§ 551.22. Criteria for performance of ambulatory surgery on pediatric patients.

In addition to the criteria in § 551.21 (relating to criteria for ambulatory surgery), the following criteria apply to the performance of ambulatory surgery on children under 18 years of age:

(1)   A child under 6 months of age may not be treated in an ASF.

(2) The medical record shall include documentation that the child's primary care provider was notified by the surgeon in advance of the performance of a procedure in an ASF and that an opinion was sought from the primary care provider regarding the appropriateness of the use of the facility for the pro- posed procedure. When an opinion from the child's primary care provider is not obtainable, the medical record shall include documentation which explains why an opinion could not be obtained.

(3) Surgical procedures on persons older than 6 months and younger than 18 years of age shall be performed only under the following conditions:

(i) Anesthesia services shall be provided by an anesthesiologist who is a graduate of an anesthesiology residency program accredited by the accreditation council for graduate medical education or its equivalent, or by a certified registered nurse anesthetist trained in pediatric anesthesia, either of whom shall have documented demonstrated historical and continuous competence in the care of these patients.

(ii) The practitioner performing the surgery shall be either board certified by or have obtained preboard certification status with the American Board of Medical Specialties, the American Osteopathic Board of Surgery, the American Board of Podiatric Surgery or the American Board of Oral and Maxillofacial Surgery.

(4) A medical professional who has successfully completed a course in advanced pediatric life support offered by the American Academy of Pediatrics and either the American College of Emergency Physicians or the American Heart Association shall be present in the facility.

Source

The provisions of this § 551.22 adopted October 22, 1999, effective November 22, 1999, 29 Pa.B. 5583.

Cross References

This section cited in 28 Pa. Code § 553.3 (relating to governing body responsibilities).

APPLICATION AND AUTHORIZATION TO OPERATE AN ASF

§ 551.31. Licensure.

(a) A Class A ASF shall meet the following criteria:

(1) A license is not required for the operation of a Class A ASF. The facility shall be accredited by the Accreditation Association for Ambulatory Health Care, the Joint Commission on the Accreditation of Health Care Organizations, the American Association for the Accreditation of Ambulatory Surgical Facilities or another Nationally recognized accrediting agency acknowledged by the Medicare Program in order to be identified as providing ambulatory surgery.

(2) A Class A ASF shall register with the Department and shall forward a copy of its accreditation survey to the Department.

(3) The Class A registration form shall request the following information, which shall also be provided to the Department by the Class A ASF on an annual basis.

(i)   A list of operative procedures proposed to be performed at the facility and the ages of the patients to be served.

(ii) The type of anesthetic proposed to be used for each operative procedure.

(iii) The facility's current accreditation survey and the designation of accreditation status by the Nationally recognized accrediting agency.

(iv) Other information the Department deems pertinent to registration requirements.

(b) A license shall be obtained to operate a freestanding Class B or Class C ASF.

(c) An ASF license shall designate the licensed facility as either a Class B or Class C.

(d) An applicant for a license to operate an ASF shall request licensure by the

Department by means of written communication which sets forth:

(1) A list of operative procedures proposed to be performed at the facility and the ages of the patients to be served.

(2) The highest level of anesthetic proposed to be used for each proposed operative procedure.

(3) The highest PS patient level proposed to receive ambulatory surgery at the facility.

(4) A statement from the applicant which may be accompanied by a writ- ten opinion from a Nationally recognized accrediting body stating the most appropriate facility Class (B or C).

(e) If a facility desires to change its classification level from a Class B enterprise to a Class C enterprise, the facility shall request and obtain a license prior to providing services to ASF Class III or PS-III patients.

(f) The Department may enter and inspect an ASF (Class A, B or C), at any time, announced or unannounced, to investigate any complaints. The Department may mandate closure of an ASF that the Department determines is providing substandard care or for any other lawful reason.

Source

The provisions of this § 551.31 amended October 22, 1999, effective November 22, 1999, 29 Pa.B. 5583. Immediately preceding text appears at serial page (251638).

Cross References

This section cited in 28 Pa. Code § 551.53 (relating to presurvey preparation).

§ 551.32. [Reserved].

Source

The provisions of this § 551.32 reserved October 22, 1999, effective November 22, 1999, 29 Pa.B. 5583. Immediately preceding text appears at serial pages (251638) to (251639).

§ 551.33. Survey.

The Department will conduct a survey to insure that the applicant is in compliance with this subpart. The survey will include an onsite inspection and review of written approvals submitted to the Department by regulatory agencies responsible for building, electric, fire and environmental safety. The Department may designate Nationally recognized accrediting agencies whose standards are at least as stringent as the Department's to perform some or all aspects of licensure surveys.

Source

The provisions of this § 551.33 amended October 22, 1999, effective November 22, 1999, 29 Pa.B. 5583. Immediately preceding text appears at serial page (251639).

§ 551.34. Licensure process.

(a) An application for the appropriate license to operate an ASF shall be made in accordance with section 807 of the act (35 P. S. § 448.807).

(b) The application form for a license to operate an ASF shall be obtained from the Department of Health, Division of Acute and Ambulatory Care Facilities, Post Office Box 90, Harrisburg, Pennsylvania 17108.

(c) Applications for renewal of a license shall be made annually on forms obtained from the Department.

(d) Applications or renewal forms shall be accompanied by a fee of $250.

Source

The provisions of this § 551.34 amended October 22, 1999, effective November 22, 1999, 29 Pa.B. 5583. Immediately preceding text appears at serial page (251639).

CONTINUING OPERATIONS

§ 551.41. Policy.

The Department will issue a license valid for 1 year to an ASF which is in compliance with this subpart.

Source

The provisions of this § 551.41 amended October 22, 1999, effective November 22, 1999, 29 Pa.B. 5583. Immediately preceding text appears at serial page (251639).

§ 551.42. [Reserved].

Source

The provisions of this § 551.42 reserved October 22, 1999, effective November 22, 1999, 29 Pa.B. 5583. Immediately preceding text appears at serial page (251639).

§ 551.43. Void license.

(a) The license of an ASF becomes automatically void when one of the fol- lowing occurs:

(1) The license term of 1 year expires.

(2) The ASF substantially changes its name or location, in which case a new license will be automatically issued upon application by an ASF if the ASF is otherwise in compliance with this subpart.

(b) If the ASF locates or relocates services at a site other than the current site or a site contiguous thereto, the ASF shall notify the Department 30 days prior to the change so that the Department may determine if a new license is necessary.

Source

The provisions of this § 551.43 amended October 22, 1999, effective November 22, 1999, 29 Pa.B. 5583. Immediately preceding text appears at serial pages (251639) to (251640).

§ 551.44. Display of license.

The current license shall be displayed in a public and conspicuous place in the ASF.

§ 551.45. Licensure information/application.

Information regarding licensure shall be completed annually on forms supplied by the Department. Both the Annual ASF Questionnaire and the Application for Licensure and other data requested by the Department shall be completed each year.

INSPECTION AND SURVEY ACTIVITIES

§ 551.51. Policy.

Representatives of the Department will annually conduct a survey of every ASF required to be licensed.

§ 551.52. ASF responsibilities.

An ASF shall comply with applicable standards which are required by Federal, State and local authorities. This includes, but is not limited to, standards at 49 Pa. Code Chapters 17, 21 and 27 (relating to State Board of Medicine—medical doctors; State Board of

Nursing; and State Board of Pharmacy) in addition to standards related to radiologic health, sanitation, food service, electric wiring and life safety code compliance. When the ASF has been inspected by another regulatory agency, it shall have available during the survey by the Department written confirmation of compliance as required by the other regulatory agency.

§ 551.53. Presurvey preparation.

Prior to an annual survey site visit of an ASF by the Department, the Department may request from the ASF documents or records of the ASF, or other information necessary for the Department to prepare for the site visit. The ASF shall provide the information requested, including a declarative statement that sets forth the information requested in § 551.31 (relating to licensure) as follows:

(1)   A list of operative procedures proposed to be performed at the facility.

(2)   The highest level of anesthetic proposed to be used for each proposed operative procedure.

(3) The highest PS patient level proposed to receive outpatient surgical treatments at the facility.

Source

The provisions of this § 551.53 amended October 22, 1999, effective November 22, 1999, 29 Pa.B. 5583. Immediately preceding text appears at serial page (251640).

Cross References

This section cited in 28 Pa. Code § 553.4 (relating to other functions).

§ 551.54. Access by the Department.

Upon presenting the official Department identification card to the ASF's per- son in charge, authorized agents of the Department will have access to the ASF to determine compliance with this subpart. The access shall include:

(1) Entry to the entire ASF premises.

(2) Inspection and examination of the facilities, records, documents and phases of operations, including those relating to compliance with Chapter 553 (relating to ownership, governance and management).

(3) Interviews of staff, employees, members of the governing body and patients.

(4) Examination of a patient, with the patient's consent.

§ 551.55. Site survey coverage.

The Department will survey on-site those aspects of the ASF as it deems necessary to fully and fairly assess the compliance of the ASF with this subpart.

§ 551.56. Documentation.

The Department will document the extent of an ASF's compliance with this subpart in at least one of the following ways:

(1) The statement of a person in charge or staff member.

(2) Documentary evidence provided by the facility.

(3) Answers by the ASF to detailed questions provided by the Department concerning the implementation of this subpart or examples of the implementation which will enable a judgment about compliance to be made.

(4) One observation by surveyors.

(5) Interviews with patients, employees or other persons or sources capable of providing reliable information to the Department.

POST SURVEY PROCEDURES

§ 551.61. Policy.

After completion of the site visit, the Department will evaluate relevant information gathered during the survey, formulate its compliance findings and determinations, and order the ASF to correct, within a specified period of time, deficiencies found.

§ 551.62. Compliance directive.

(a) If there is noncompliance with this subpart, the Department will notify the ASF in writing of deficiencies and will direct the officers governing or managing the ASF to take corrective action as the Department directs or to submit a plan of correction, or to do both, within the time specified by the Department. In its compliance directive and request for plan of correction, the Department will state its findings and the reasons for its determination.

(b) The ASF shall be presumed to be in compliance with provisions of this subpart for which the compliance directive does not cite a deficiency.

§ 551.63. Submission of plan of correction.

A plan of correction shall be submitted to the Department within 30 days of receipt of written notification by the Department. The plan shall be attested to by the signature of the chairman of the governing body or the person in charge. The plan of correction shall be submitted to the governing body as a whole for its review at its regular meeting.

§ 551.64. Content of plan of correction.

A plan of correction shall address deficiencies cited in the compliance directive of the Department. The plan shall state specifically what corrective action is to be taken, by whom and when.

§ 551.65. Public inspection of compliance documents.

Copies of compliance directives and plans of correction will be kept readily available by the Department in appropriate regional offices for the purpose of public inspection, examination and duplication at a reasonable cost. An ASF shall make available a current copy of these documents for inspection and examination.

CONTINUING SURVEILLANCE

§ 551.71. Unannounced surveys.

Whenever the Department has received a complaint or has other reasonable grounds to believe that a deficiency exists, the Department may without notice to the ASF investigate, inspect or survey the facility, or portion of the ASF to which the alleged deficiency relates.

ISSUANCE OF LICENSE

§ 551.81. Principle.

The Department will issue an ASF license to a facility which complies with this subpart. The license will reflect the regular, provisional or limited status and the classification assigned to the ASF. The license applies only to the designated facility.

Source

The provisions of this § 551.81 amended October 22, 1999, effective November 22, 1999, 29 Pa.B. 5583. Immediately preceding text appears at serial page (251642).

§ 551.82. Regular license.

(a) The Department will issue a regular license to an ASF when that ASF is in compliance with section 808 of the act (35 P. S. § 448.808) and is in full or substantial compliance with this subpart.

(b) As used in subsection (a) "substantial compliance" means:

(1) Deficiencies are, individually and in combined effect, of a minor nature so that neither the deficiencies nor efforts toward their correction will do one of the following:

(i) Interfere with or adversely affect normal ASF operations. (ii) Adversely affect a patient's health or safety.

(iii) Exceed the assigned classification of the ASF.

(2) The ASF has adopted a plan of correction approved by the Department.

Source

The provisions of this § 551.82 amended October 22, 1999, effective November 22, 1999, 29 Pa.B. 5583. Immediately preceding text appears at serial pages (251642) to (251643).

Cross References

This section cited in 28 Pa. Code § 551.91 (relating to grounds); 28 Pa. Code § 551.92 (relating to modification of license); and 28 Pa. Code § 551.101 (relating to policy).

§ 551.83. Provisional license.

(a)   The Department may issue a provisional license if:

(1) There are numerous deficiencies or a serious specific deficiency in compliance with applicable statutes, ordinances or regulations.

(2) The ASF is taking appropriate steps to correct the deficiencies in accordance with a plan of correction submitted by the ASF and agreed upon by the Department.

(3) There is no cyclical pattern of deficiencies over a period of 2 or more years. A cyclical pattern is one where an ASF is alternately in and out of substantial or full compliance, which is corrected only when actively supervised by the Department.

(b) A provisional license is valid for a specific time period of no more than 6 months.

(c)   A provisional license may be renewed no more than three times.

Source

The provisions of this § 551.83 amended October 22, 1999, effective November 22, 1999, 29 Pa.B. 5583. Immediately preceding text appears at serial page (251643).

Cross References

This section cited in 28 Pa. Code § 551.91 (relating to grounds); and 28 Pa. Code § 551.92 (relating to modification of license).

REFUSAL OR REVOCATION

§ 551.91. Grounds.

(a) The Department may refuse to issue a license for one or more of the following reasons:

(1)   The health care provider is not a responsible person.

(2) The place to be used as an ASF is not adequately constructed, equipped, maintained and operated to safely and efficiently render the services offered.

(3) The ASF does not provide safe and efficient services which are adequate for the care, treatment and comfort of the patients or residents of the facility.

(4)   There is not substantial compliance with this subpart.

(b) The Department may refuse to renew a license, or may suspend or revoke or limit a license for all or a portion of an ASF, or for a particular service offered by an ASF, or may suspend admissions for any of the following reasons:

(1) Serious violation of or noncompliance with the act or with this subpart except when the ASF is in compliance or substantial compliance as defined in

§ 551.82 (relating to regular license) or otherwise meets the conditions in § 551.83 (relating to provisional license). A serious violation is one which poses a significant threat to the health of a patient.

(2) Failure to submit a plan of correction when required to do so, or failure, by the holder of a provisional license, to correct a deficiency under a plan of correction, unless the Department approves an extension or modification of the plan of correction.

(3) Incompetence, negligence or misconduct in operating the ASF, or in providing services to patients.

(4) Fraud or deceit in obtaining or attempting to obtain a license.
(5) Lending, borrowing or using the license of another ASF.

(6) Knowingly aiding or abetting the improper granting of a license.

(7) Mistreating or abusing individuals cared for by the ASF.

(8) The existence of a cyclical pattern of deficiencies over a period of 2 or more years. A cyclical pattern means an ASF is alternately in and out of full or substantial compliance, which is corrected only when actively supervised by the Department.

(9) Serious violation of the laws relating to Medical Assistance or Medicare reimbursement.

(10) Providing services exceeding the scope of the classification assigned in the license.

Source

The provisions of this § 551.91 amended October 22, 1999, effective November 22, 1999, 29 Pa.B. 5583. Immediately preceding text appears at serial pages (251643) to (251644).

§ 551.92. Modification of license.

The Department may modify a license by substituting a provisional license for a regular license if the Department determines that the ASF is not in compliance or substantial compliance as defined in § 551.82 (relating to regular license) but the ASF otherwise meets the requirements of § 551.83 (relating to provisional license).

§ 551.93. Notice.

(a) If the Department proposes to revoke, modify, limit or refuse to issue or renew a license or to issue a provisional license, or to suspend admissions or to levy a civil penalty against the ASF, it will give written notice to the ASF by certified mail.

(b) Written notice will specify the reasons for the proposed action of the Department and will notify the ASF of its right to a hearing. The order will specify the time within which a request of the ASF for a hearing shall be filed with the Health Policy Board.

Source

The provisions of this § 551.93 amended October 22, 1999, effective November 22, 1999, 29 Pa.B. 5583. Immediately preceding text appears at serial page (251644).

§ 551.101. Policy.

CORRECTION OF DEFICIENCY

If an ASF notifies the Department that it has completed a plan of correction and corrected its deficiencies, the Department will conduct a survey to ascertain completion of the plan of correction.

Upon finding full or substantial compliance, as defined in §
551.82(b) (relating to a regular license), the Department will issue a
regular license.

HEARINGS

§ 551.111. Hearings relating to licensure.

Hearings relating to licensure, including the issuance of a
provisional license, or the suspension of admissions, will be
conducted by the Health Policy Board, under 37 Pa. Code Chapter
197 (relating to practice and procedure).

Source

The provisions of this § 551.111 amended October 22, 1999, effective
November 22, 1999, 29 Pa.B. 5583. Immediately preceding text
appears at serial page (251645).

§§ 551.121—551.123. [Reserved].

Source

The provisions of these §§ 551.121—551.123 reserved October 22,
1999, effective November 22, 1999, 29 Pa.B. 5583. Immediately
preceding text appears at serial page (251645).

CHAPTER 553.

OWNERSHIP, GOVERNANCE AND MANAGEMENT

Authority

The provisions of this Chapter 553 issued under Chapter 8 of the

Health Care Facilities Act (35 P. S. §§ 448.801a—448.820), specifically sections 448.801a and 448.803; and section 2102(a) and (g) of The Administrative Code of 1929 (71 P. S. § 532(a) and (g)), unless otherwise noted.

Source

The provisions of this Chapter 553 adopted January 23, 1987, effective March 25, 1987, 17 Pa.B. 376, unless otherwise noted.

Cross References

This chapter cited in 28 Pa. Code § 551.54 (relating to access by the Department).

GOVERNING BODY

§ 553.1. Principle.

There shall be an organized governing body or designated person vested with ownership who shall assume the full legal authority and responsibility for the conduct of the ASF.

§ 553.2. Ownership.

(a) The owner of the ASF may be an individual, partnership, association, a corporation or a combination thereof.

(b) A complete list of the names and addresses of owners, directors, officers and managers shall be submitted with the application.

(c) Owners shall be considered any person who has a direct or indirect equity interest in the facility of 5% or more, including shareholders and partners.

(d) A physically noncontiguous branch of the ASF shall meet the requirements for licensure and shall be independently licensed.

Source

The provisions of this § 553.2 amended October 22, 1999, effective November 22, 1999, 29 Pa.B. 5583. Immediately preceding text appears at serial page (247506).

§ 553.3. Governing body responsibilities.

Governing body responsibilities include:

(1) Conforming to applicable Federal, State and local law. (2) Determining the goals and objectives of the ASF.

(3) Assuring that facilities and personnel are adequate and appropriate to carry out the goals and objectives.

(4) Establishing an organizational structure and specifying functional relationships among the various components of the ASF.

(5) Adopting bylaws or similar rules and regulations for the orderly development and management of the ASF, which:

(i) Describe the authority delegated to the person in charge and to the medical staff.

(ii) Require the governing body to review and approve the bylaws, or similar rules and regulations, of the medical staff.

(6) Adopting policies or procedures necessary for the orderly conduct of the ASF.

(7) Assuring that the quality of care is evaluated and that identified problems are appropriately addressed.

(8) Establishing personnel policies and practices which adequately support sound patient care to include the following:

(i) Require the employment of personnel with qualifications commensurate with a job's responsibilities and authority, including appropriate licensure and certification.

(ii) Applicants for positions requiring a licensed person shall be hired only after obtaining verification of their licenses, records of education and written references.

(iii) Personnel records shall include current information relative to periodic work performance evaluations.

(iv) Compliance with Occupational Safety and Health Administration

(OSHA) Universal Precautions for prevention of transmission of diseases.

(v) Written job descriptions shall exist for each type of job in the ASF. (vi) Compliance with Federal and State regulations including, The Americans with Disabilities Act of 1990 (42 U.S.C.A. §§ 12101—12213), civil rights and OSHA regulations.

(9) Reviewing legal and ethical matters concerning the ASF including the reports and disposition of unusual incidents.

(10) Maintaining effective communication throughout the ASF.

(11) Establishing a system of financial management and accountability that includes an audit appropriate for the ASF.

(12) Establishing a procedure for implementing, disseminating and enforcing a patient's bill of rights in compliance with § 553.13

(relating to procedures for distribution).

(13) Approving major contracts or arrangements affecting the medical care provided under its auspices, including those concerning:

(i) The employment for contractual arrangements with practitioners and others providing direct patient care.

(ii) The provision of all treatment related services including, radiology, medical laboratory, pathology, anesthesia and pharmaceutical services.

(iii) The provision of care by other health care organizations.

(iv) The provision of education to students and postgraduate trainees. (14) Formulating long-range plans in accordance with the goals and objectives of the ASF.

(15) Operating the ASF without limitation because of age, race, creed, color, sex, national origin, religion, handicap or disability.

(16) Assuring that at least one medical professional in the facility when patients are present is currently and on an ongoing basis certified in advanced cardiac life support, or its successor. If a pediatric patient is present in the facility, the certification of the medical professional shall be in advanced pediatric life support as defined in § 551.22(4) (relating to criteria for performance of ambulatory surgery on pediatric patients).

Source

The provisions of this § 553.3 adopted January 23, 1987, effective March 25, 1987, 17 Pa.B. 376; amended July 21, 1989, effective July 22, 1989, 19 Pa.B. 3105; amended October 22, 1999, effective

November 22, 1999, 29 Pa.B. 5583. Immediately preceding text appears at serial pages (247506) to (247508).

§ 553.4. Other functions.

(a) The governing body shall meet at least annually and keep minutes or other records necessary for the orderly conduct of the ASF.

(b) If the governing body elects, appoints or employs officers and administrators to carry out its directives, the authority, responsibility and functions of the positions shall be defined.

(c) If the governing body is comprised of two or more members, and if the majority of those members are practitioners, the governing body, either directly or by delegation, shall make—based on evidence of the education, training and current competence—initial appointments, reappointments and assignment or curtailment of clinical privileges of the practitioners.

(d) If the governing body is comprised of only one member, or if a majority of the members of the governing body are not practitioners, the ASF bylaws or similar rules and regulations shall specify a procedure for establishing medical review by practitioners for the purpose of recommending to the governing body for its approval based on evidence of the education, training and current competence—initial appointments, reappointments and assignment or curtailment of clinical privileges of the practitioners.

(e) If students and postgraduate trainees are present in the facility, their role and functions shall be defined.

(f) The governing body shall ensure that personnel are provided with continuing education which is relevant to their responsibilities within the organization.

(g) The governing body shall ensure that the licensee provides to the Department, the documents under § 551.53 (relating to presurvey preparation).

(h) The governing body shall appoint a medical director who shall be board certified by an American Board of Medical Specialties recognized board or the dental, podiatric or osteopathic equivalent. The governing body may appoint an interim director during the period of time between the departure of a director and the selection of a new director.

(1)   The interim director shall be a physician who is able to demonstrate qualifications acceptable to the medical staff of the ASF and to the Department. (2)   If the interim director is not board certified, the Department will specify the maximum period of time for which the interim director may serve.

Source

The provisions of this § 553.4 amended October 22, 1999, effective November 22, 1999, 29 Pa.B. 5583. Immediately preceding text appears at serial page (247508).

Cross References

This section cited in 28 Pa. Code § 551.3 (relating to definitions).

PATIENT'S BILL OF RIGHTS

§ 553.11. Purpose.

The purpose of §§ 553.11—553.13 (relating to patient's bill of rights) is to promote the interests and well-being of the patients of ambulatory surgical facilities subject to this subpart even in those instances where the interests of the patients may be in opposition to the interests of the ASF. It is the policy of the Department that the interests of patients be protected by a patient's bill of rights. Nothing in §§ 553.11—553.13 is intended to serve as evidence of a standard of reasonable conduct for the purpose of determining civil liability between providers and consumers of health services. The ASF has the right to expect the patient to fulfill patient responsibilities as may be stated in the ASF's rules affecting patient care and conduct.

§ 553.12. Implementation.

(a) The ASF governing body shall establish a patient's bill of rights not less in substance and coverage than the minimal patient's bill of rights provided by subsection (b).

(b) The following are minimal provisions for the patient's bill of rights:

(1)   A patient has the right to respectful care given by competent personnel.

(2)   A patient has the right, upon request, to be given the name of his attending practitioner, the names of all other practitioners directly participating in his care and the names and functions of other health care persons having direct contact with the patient.

(3) A patient has the right to consideration of privacy concerning his own medical care program. Case discussion, consultation, examination and treatment are considered confidential and shall be conducted discreetly.

(4) A patient has the right to have records pertaining to his medical

care treated as confidential except as otherwise provided by law or third party contractual arrangements.

(5) A patient has the right to know what ASF rules and regulations apply to his conduct as a patient.

(6) The patient has the right to expect emergency procedures to be implemented without unnecessary delay.

(7) The patient has the right to good quality care and high professional standards that are continually maintained and reviewed.

(8) The patient has the right to full information in layman's terms, concerning diagnosis, treatment and prognosis, including information about alternative treatments and possible complications. When it is not medically advisable to give the information to the patient, the information shall be given on his behalf to the responsible person.

(9) Except for emergencies, the practitioner shall obtain the necessary informed consent prior to the start of a procedure. Informed consent is defined in section 103 of the Health Care Services Malpractice Act (40 P. S. § 1301.103).

(10) A patient or, if the patient is unable to give informed consent, a responsible person, has the right to be advised when a practitioner is considering the patient as a part of a medical care research program or donor program, and the patient, or responsible person, shall give informed consent prior to actual participation in the program. A patient, or responsible person, may refuse to continue in a program to which he has previously given informed consent.

(11) A patient has the right to refuse drugs or procedures, to the

extent per mitted by statute, and a practitioner shall inform the patient of the medical consequences of the patient's refusal of drugs or procedures.

(12) A patient has the right to medical and nursing services without dis crimination based upon age, race, color, religion, sex, national origin, handicap, disability or source of payment.

(13) The patient who does not speak English shall have access, where possible, to an interpreter.

(14) The ASF shall provide the patient, or patient designee, upon request, access to the information contained in his medical records, unless access is specifically restricted by the attending practitioner for medical reasons.

(15) The patient has the right to expect good management techniques to be implemented within the ASF. These techniques shall make effective use of the time of the patient and avoid the personal discomfort of the patient.

(16) When an emergency occurs and a patient is transferred to another facility, the responsible person shall be notified. The institution to which the patient is to be transferred shall be notified prior to the patient's transfer.

(17) The patient has the right to examine and receive a detailed explanation of his bill.

(18) A patient has the right to expect that the ASF will provide information for continuing health care requirements following discharge and the means for meeting them.

(19) A patient has the right to be informed of his rights at the time

of admission.

Cross Reference

This section cited in 28 Pa. Code § 553.11 (relating to purpose).

§ 553.13. Procedures for distribution.

The ASF shall develop procedures to inform each patient of his rights. Copies of the ASF's patient's bill of rights shall be made generally available through one of the following ways:

(1) Prominent displays in appropriate locations in addition to copies available upon request.

(2) Provision of a copy to each patient or responsible party upon admission.

Cross References

This section cited in 28 Pa. Code § 553.3 (relating to governing body responsibilities); and 28 Pa. Code § 553.11 (relating to purpose).

ADMISSION, TRANSFER AND DISCHARGE

§ 553.21. Principle.

(a) The ASF shall have written policies for the admission, discharge, transfer and proper referral of patients.

(b) The ASF may not provide beds or other accommodations for an overnight stay of patients.

(c) A patient shall be discharged in a conscious and coherent condition and able to maintain vital life functions or shall be transferred to a hospital.

(d) A patient shall be discharged only with appropriate discharge instructions under § 555.24 (relating to postoperative care).

Source

The provisions of this § 553.21 amended October 22, 1999, effective November 22, 1999, 29 Pa.B. 5583. Immediately preceding text appears at serial page (247511).

§ 553.22. Admission criteria.

The governing body, with the advice of and in conjunction with the medical staff, shall establish medical criteria for admissions under § 555.22(a) (relating to preoperative care). Medical criteria shall be congruent with the assigned ASF class level stated on the facility license.

Source

The provisions of this § 553.22 amended October 22, 1999, effective November 22, 1999, 29 Pa.B. 5583. Immediately preceding text appears at serial page (247511).

§ 553.23. Discharge by transfer.

A patient may not be transferred to another medical facility unless prior arrangements for admission have been made. Clinical records of sufficient con tent to insure continuity of care shall accompany the patient.

§ 553.24. Discharge of a minor or incompetent patient.

An individual who cannot legally consent to his own care shall be discharged only to the custody of parents, legal guardian, person standing in loco parentis or another responsible party unless otherwise directed by the parent or guardian or court of competent jurisdiction. If the parent or guardian directs that discharge be made otherwise, he shall so state in writing and the statement shall become a part of the permanent medical record of the patient.

§ 553.25. Discharge criteria.

A patient may only be discharged from an ASF if the following physical status criteria are met:

(1) Vital signs. Blood pressure, heart rate, temperature and respiratory rate are within the normal range for the patient's age or at preoperative levels for that patient.

(2) Activity. The patient has regained preoperative mobility without assistance or syncope, or function at the patient's usual level considering limitations imposed by the surgical procedure.

(3) Mental status. The patient is awake, alert or functions at the patient's preoperative mental status.

(4) Pain. The patient's pain can be effectively controlled with medication.

(5) Bleeding. Bleeding is controlled and consistent with that expected from the surgical procedure.

(6) Nausea/vomiting. Minimal nausea or vomiting is controlled and consistent with that expected from the surgical procedure.

Source

The provisions of this § 553.25 adopted October 22, 1999, effective November 22, 1999, 29 Pa.B. 5583.

MANAGEMENT AND ADMINISTRATION OF OPERATIONS

§ 553.31. Administrative responsibilities.

(a) A fulltime person in charge shall be appointed who has authority and responsibility for the operation of the ASF at all times. Qualifications, authority, responsibilities and duties of the person in charge shall be defined in a written statement adopted by the governing body.

(b) Administrative policies, procedures and controls shall be established, documented and implemented to assure the orderly and efficient management of the ASF.

Source

The provisions of this § 553.31 amended October 22, 1999, effective November 22, 1999, 29 Pa.B. 5583. Immediately preceding text appears at serial pages (247511) to (247512). [Next page is 555-1.]

CHAPTER 555. MEDICAL STAFF

Authority

The provisions of this Chapter 555 issued under Chapter 8 of the Health Care Facilities Act (35 P. S. §§ 448.801a—448.820), specifically sections 448.801a and 448.803; section 2102(a) and (g) of

The Administrative Code of 1929 (71 P. S. § 532(a) and (g)), unless otherwise noted.

Source

The provisions of this Chapter 555 adopted January 23, 1987, effective March 25, 1987, 17 Pa.B. 376, unless otherwise noted.

MEDICAL STAFF

§ 555.1. Principle.

There shall be an organized medical staff which is accountable to the governing body and which has responsibility for the quality of medical care provided to patients and for the ethical conduct and professional practice of its members and other practitioners who have been granted clinical privileges in the ASF.

Cross References

This section cited in 28 Pa. Code § 551.3 (relating to definitions).

§ 555.2. Medical staff membership.

A member of the medical staff shall be qualified for membership and the exercise of clinical privileges granted to him. The governing body of the ASF, after considering the recommendations of the medical staff, may grant clinical privileges to qualified, licensed practitioners in accordance with their training, experience and demonstrated competence and judgment. Members of the medical staff and others granted clinical privileges shall currently hold licenses to practice in this Commonwealth.

Cross References

This section cited in 28 Pa. Code § 551.3 (relating to definitions).

§ 555.3. Requirements for membership and privileges.

(a) To receive favorable recommendation for appointment, or reappointment, members of the medical staff shall always act in a manner consistent with the highest ethical standards and levels of professional competence.

(b) Privileges granted shall reflect the results of peer review or utilization review programs, or both, specific to ambulatory surgery.

(c) Privileges granted shall be commensurate with an individual's qualifications, experience and present capabilities.

(d) Granting of clinical privileges shall follow established policies and procedures in the bylaws or similar rules and regulations. The procedures shall provide the following:

(1) A written record of the application, which includes the scope of privileges sought and granted. The delineation "clinical privileges" shall address the administration of anesthesia.

(2) A review, summarized on record with appropriate documentation, of the qualifications of the applicant.

(e) Reappraisal and reappointment shall be required of every member of the medical staff at regular intervals no longer than every 2 years.

(f) The governing body shall request and consider reports from the National Practitioner Data Bank on each practitioner who requests privileges.

Source

The provisions of this § 555.3 amended October 22, 1999, effective November 22, 1999, 29 Pa.B. 5583. Immediately preceding text appears at serial page (256562).

Cross References

This section cited in 28 Pa. Code § 551.3 (relating to definitions).

§ 555.4. Clinical activities and duties of physician assistants and certified registered nurse practitioners.

(a) If the ASF assigns patient care responsibilities to physician assistants and nurse practitioners, the medical staff shall have established policies and procedures approved by the governing body, for overseeing and evaluating their clinical activities. The training, experience and demonstrated current competence of physician assistants and nurse practitioners shall be commensurate with their duties and responsibilities.

(b) Physician assistants shall perform within the limits established by the medical staff and consistent with the Medical Practice Act of 1985 (63 P. S. §§ 422.1—422.45) and the Osteopathic Medical Practice Act (63 P. S. §§ 261—271). Certified registered nurse practitioners shall perform within the limits established by the medical staff and consistent with the Professional Nursing Law (63P. S. §§ 211—225.5) and the joint regulations of the State Boards of Medicine and Nursing.

(c) Physician assistants and nurse practitioners shall be licensed or certified as applicable.

Source

The provisions of this § 555.4 amended October 22, 1999, effective November 22, 1999, 29 Pa.B. 5583. Immediately preceding text appears at serial page (256563).

MEDICAL ORDERS

§ 555.11. Written orders.

(a) Medication or treatment shall be administered by authorized persons to administer drugs and medications only upon written and signed orders of a practitioner acting within the scope of the practitioner's license.

(b) Physician assistants and certified registered nurse practitioners may write orders for medication or treatment in accordance with their legally authorized scope of practice and policies and procedures of the ASF.

(c) Written orders may be issued by facsimile transmission.

Source

The provisions of this § 555.11 amended October 22, 1999, effective November 22, 1999, 29 Pa.B. 5583. Immediately preceding text appears at serial page (256563).

§ 555.12. Oral orders.

Oral orders for medication or treatment shall be accepted only under urgent circumstances when it is impractical for the orders to be given in written manner by the responsible practitioner. Oral orders shall be administered in accordance with § 555.13 (relating to administration of drugs) only by personnel qualified by their professional license or certification issued by the Commonwealth and according to medical staff bylaws or rules, who shall document the orders in the proper place in the medical record of the patient. The order shall include the date, time and full signature of the person taking the order and shall be countersigned by a practitioner within 48 hours of the order. If the practitioner is not the attending physician, the practitioner shall be authorized by the attending physician and shall be knowledgeable about the patient's condition.

Countersignatures may be received by facsimile transmission.

Source

The provisions of this § 555.12 amended October 22, 1999, effective November 22, 1999, 29 Pa.B. 5583. Immediately preceding text appears at serial page (256563).

§ 555.13. Administration of drugs.

Drugs shall be administered only upon the proper order of a practitioner acting within the scope of the practitioner's license and authorized according to medical staff bylaws, rules and regulations. Drugs shall be administered directly by a practitioner qualified according to medical staff bylaws, rules and regulations or by a professional nurse or by a licensed practical nurse with pharmacy training. Physician assistants and certified registered nurse practitioners shall be permitted to administer drugs within their authorized scope of practice. Further policies on the administration of drugs shall be established by the medical staff in conjunction with pharmaceutical services or personnel.

Source

The provisions of this § 555.13 adopted October 22, 1999, effective November 22, 1999, 29 Pa.B. 5583.

SURGICAL SERVICES

§ 555.21. Surgical procedures.

Procedures performed in the ASF are limited to procedures that are approved by the governing body, upon the recommendation of the medical staff and congruent with ASF classification as stated on its ASF license.

Source

The provisions of this § 555.21 amended October 22, 1999, effective November 22, 1999, 29 Pa.B. 5583. Immediately preceding text appears at serial page (256563).

§ 555.22. Preoperative care.

(a) Pertinent medical histories and physical examinations, and supplemental information regarding drug sensitivities shall be documented the day of surgery or one of the following:

(1) If medical evaluation, examination and referral are made from a private practitioner's office, hospital or clinic, pertinent records thereof shall be available and made part of the patient's clinical record at the time the patient is registered and admitted to the ASF. This information is considered valid only if the evaluation was performed no more than 30 days prior to date of surgery.

(2) A practitioner shall examine the patient immediately before surgery to evaluate the risk of anesthesia and of the procedure to be performed. The information shall be clearly documented in the medical record.

(b) A written statement indicating informed consent, obtained by the practitioner, and signed by the patient, or responsible person, for the performance of the specific procedures shall be procured and made part of the patient's clinical record. It shall contain a statement which evidences the appropriateness of the proposed surgery, as well as any alternative treatments discussed with the patient. It shall also identify any practitioner who will participate in the surgery.

(c) Written instructions for preoperative procedures, which have been approved by the medical staff, shall be given to the patient or responsible person, and shall include:

(1) Applicable restrictions upon food and drink before surgery.

(2) Special preparations to be made by the patient.

(3) The required proximity of the patient to the ASF for a specific time following surgery, if applicable.

(4) An understanding that the patient may require admission to the hospital in the event of medical need.

(5) Upon discharge of a patient who has received sedation or general anesthesia, a responsible person shall be available to escort the patient home. With respect to patients who receive local or regional anesthesia, a medical decision shall be made regarding whether these patients require a responsible person to escort them home.

(d) Preoperative diagnostic studies, if performed, shall be evaluated, annotated, signed and entered into the patient's medical record before surgery.

(e) Prior to the administration of anesthesia, it is the responsibility of the primary operating surgeon and the person administering anesthesia to properly identify the patient and the procedure to be performed and to document this identification in the patient's medical record. This procedure shall be in written policies designating the mechanism to be used to identify each surgical patient.

Source

The provisions of this § 555.22 amended October 22, 1999, effective

November 22, 1999, 29 Pa.B. 5583. Immediately preceding text appears at serial pages (256563) to (256564).

Cross References

This section cited in 28 Pa. Code § 553.22 (relating to admission criteria); and 28 Pa. Code § 555.24 (relating to post-operative care).

§ 555.23. Operative care.

(a) Approved surgical procedures shall be performed only by a qualified physician, dentist or podiatrist within the limits of the practitioner's defined specific practice privileges. Physician assistants and certified registered nurse practitioners may be permitted to assist in the performance of surgical procedures in accordance with their legally authorized scope of practice and the policies and procedures of the ASF.

(b) Tissues and exudates removed during a surgical procedure shall be properly labeled and sent to a laboratory for examination by a pathologist. The specimen shall be accompanied by pertinent clinical information, including its source and the preoperative and postoperative surgical diagnosis. The pathologist's signed report of the examination shall be made a part of the patient's medical record. Certain tissues and exudates may be exempt from laboratory examination. The exemptions shall be those that are consistent with current medical practices and are in writing and approved by the governing body.

(c) An ASF shall be prepared to initiate immediate onsite resuscitation or other appropriate response to an emergency which may be associated with procedures performed there.

(d) The ASF shall have an effective procedure for the immediate transfer to a hospital of patients requiring emergency medical care beyond the capabilities of the ASF.

(e) The ASF shall have a written transfer agreement with a hospital which has emergency and surgical services available, or physicians performing surgery in the ASF shall have admitting privileges at a hospital in close proximity to the ASF, to which patients may be transferred.

(f) There shall be a written agreement in effect with an ambulance service staffed by certified EMT personnel, for the safe transfer of a patient to a hospital in an emergency situation, or as the need arises.

Source

The provisions of this § 555.23 amended October 22, 1999, effective November 22, 1999, 29 Pa.B. 5583. Immediately preceding text appears at serial pages (256564) to (256565).

§ 555.24. Postoperative care.

(a) The findings and techniques of an operation shall be accurately and completely written or dictated immediately after the procedure by the practitioner medical staff member who performed the operation. If a physician assistant or certified registered nurse practitioner performed part of the operation, the findings and techniques of the procedure shall be accurately recorded and the report shall be countersigned by the medical staff member. This description shall become a part of the patient's medical record.

(b) A patient who has received anesthesia shall be observed in the facility by a registered nurse, physician assistant or a practitioner for a period of time which is sufficient to ensure that no immediate postoperative complications are present.

(c) Patients in whom a complication is known or suspected to have occurred during or after the performance of a surgical procedure shall be informed of the condition and arrangements made for treatment of the complication. In the event of admission to an inpatient facility, a summary of care given in the ASF concerning the suspected complication shall accompany the patient.

(d) A medical professional certified in advanced cardiac life support shall be present until patients operated on that day have been discharged from the facility. If a patient receives general anesthesia, regional anesthesia or IV sedation, an anesthetist shall remain present until that patient has been discharged from the facility.

(e) Patients shall be discharged in the company of a responsible person, if one is deemed to be necessary under § 555.22(c)(5) (relating to preoperative care).

(f) Protocols approved by the medical staff shall be established for instructing patients in self-care after surgery including written instructions which, at a minimum, include the following:

(1) The symptoms of complications associated with procedures performed.

(2) An explanation of prescribed drug regime including directions for use of medications.

(3) The limitations and restrictions on activities of the patient, if necessary.

(4) A specific telephone number to be used by the patient, if a complication or question arises.

(5)   A date for follow-up or return visit after the performance of the surgical procedure.

(6)   Instructions on the care of dressing and wounds.

(7)   Instructions on dietary limitations.

(g) Patients shall be discharged only on the written signed order of a practitioner.

Source

The provisions of this § 555.24 amended October 22, 1999, effective November 22, 1999, 29 Pa.B. 5583. Immediately preceding text appears at serial page (256565).

Cross References

This section cited in 28 Pa. Code § 553.21 (relating to principle).

ANESTHESIA SERVICES

§ 555.31. Principle.

 (a) Anesthesia services provided in the facility are limited to those techniques that are approved by the governing body upon the recommendation of qualified medical staff. They shall be limited to those techniques appropriate to the assigned classification per ASF license.

(b) The governing body shall define the degree of supervision required and the scope of responsibilities delegated to anesthesiologists, certified registered nurse anesthetists and dentist anesthetists, as well as the corresponding responsibilities of supervising physicians.

The provisions of this § 555.31 amended October 22, 1999, effective November 22, 1999, 29 Pa.B. 5583. Immediately preceding text appears at serial page (256566).

§ 555.32. Administration of anesthesia.

(a) Anesthetics shall be administered by anesthesiologists and certified registered nurse anesthetists and dentist anesthetists, or practitioners as defined in § 551.3 (relating to definitions).

(b) If a nonphysician administers the anesthesia, the anesthetist shall be under the overall direction of an anesthesiologist or a physician or dentist who is present in the ASF.

(c) The Director of Anesthesia Services shall be responsible for designating the physician or dentist who will be responsible for the overall direction of the anesthetist.

Source

The provisions of this § 555.32 amended October 22, 1999, effective November 22, 1999, 29 Pa.B. 5583. Immediately preceding text appears at serial page (256566).

§ 555.33. Anesthesia policies and procedures.

(a) In ASFs where an anesthesiologist is present, the anesthesiologist shall be designated the Director of Anesthesia Services and shall be responsible for directing the anesthesia services and establishing the general policies and procedures for the administration of anesthesia in the ASF which shall be approved by the governing body.

(b) In ASFs where there is no anesthesiologist, the governing body shall designate a physician or dentist to function as the Director of Anesthesia Services, who shall be responsible for directing the anesthesia services and establishing the general policies and procedures for the administration of anesthesia in the ASF which shall be approved by the governing body.

(c) Policies and procedures shall be developed for anesthesia services and shall include the following:

(1)   Education, training and supervision of personnel.

(2)   Responsibilities of nonphysician anesthetists.

(3)   Responsibilities of supervising physicians or dentists.

(d) Anesthesia procedures shall provide at least the following:

(1) A patient requiring anesthesia shall have a pre-anesthesia evaluation by a practitioner, with appropriate documentation of pertinent information regarding the choice of anesthesia.

(2) A review and documentation shall be made of the condition of the patient immediately prior to induction of anesthesia, including pertinent laboratory findings, time of administration and dosage of preanesthesia medications.

(3)   Prior to beginning the administration of anesthesia, the anesthetist shall check equipment to be used in administration of anesthetic agents. An anesthetic gas machine in anesthetizing areas shall have a pin-index safety system.

(4) Following the procedure for which anesthesia was administered; the anesthetist shall remain with the patient as long as necessary to insure safe transport to the recovery area and shall

advise personnel responsible for post- anesthetic care of the condition of the patient.

(5) A patient receiving anesthesia shall have an anesthetic record maintained. This shall include a record of vital signs and all events taking place during the induction of, maintenance of and emergence from anesthesia, including the dosage and duration of anesthetic agents, other drugs and intra- venous fluids.

(6) Intraoperative physiologic monitoring shall include the following at a minimum:

(i)   The use of oxygen saturation by pulse oximetry.

(ii) The use of End Tidal CO_2 monitoring during endotracheal anesthesia.

(iii) The use of EKG monitoring.

(iv) The use of blood pressure monitoring.

(7) A patient may not receive general anesthesia unless one or more additional health care professionals besides the one performing the surgery, are present, one of whom is trained in the administration of anesthesia.

(8) Before discharge from the ASF, a patient shall be evaluated for proper anesthesia recovery by an anesthetist, the operating room surgeon, anesthesiologist or dentist. Depending on the type of anesthesia and length of surgery, the postoperative check shall include at least the following:

(i)   Level of activity. (ii)   Respirations.

(iii) Blood pressure.

(iv) Level of consciousness.

(v) Oxygen saturation by pulse oximetry.

Source

The provisions of this § 555.33 amended October 22, 1999, effective November 22, 1999, 29 Pa.B.

5583. Immediately preceding text appears at serial pages (256566) to (256567).

§ 555.34. Development and review of safety regulations.

Regulations governing procedures to assure the safety of anesthetics and other medical gases shall be developed, approved and reviewed by appropriate representatives of the medical staff and of the governing body.

§ 555.35. Safety regulations.

(a) Appropriate precautions shall be taken to ensure the safe administration of anesthetic and other medical gas agents, in accordance with the latest edition of NFPA Code 56G, and other applicable NFPA Codes as required.

(b) The machines used for anesthesia shall have at least one annual function testing by technicians with appropriate training and a log of this testing and out- comes shall be maintained.

Source

The provisions of this § 555.35 amended October 22, 1999, effective November 22, 1999, 29 Pa.B. 5583. Immediately preceding text appears at serial page (256567).

CHAPTER 557.

QUALITY ASSURANCE AND IMPROVEMENT

Authority

The provisions of this Chapter 557 issued under Chapter 8 of the Health Care Facilities Act (35 P. S. §§ 448.801a—448.820), specifically sections 448.801a and 448.803; and section 2102(a) and (g) of The Administrative Code of 1929 (71 P. S. § 532(a) and (g)), unless otherwise noted.

Source

The provisions of this Chapter 557 adopted January 23, 1987, effective March 25, 1987, 17 Pa.B. 376, unless otherwise noted.

§ 557.1. Policy.

The ASF, with active participation of the medical and nursing staff, shall con- duct an ongoing quality assurance and improvement program designed to objectively and systematically monitor and evaluate the quality and appropriateness of patient care, pursue opportunities to improve patient care and resolve identified problems.

Source

The provisions of this § 557.1 amended October 22, 1999, effective November 22, 1999, 29 Pa.B. 5583. Immediately preceding text appears at serial page (256569).

§ 557.2. Plan.

(a) The ASF shall have a written plan for the quality assurance and improvement program that describes the program's objectives, organization, scope and mechanisms for overseeing the effectiveness of monitoring, evaluation and problem solving activities.

(b) The written plan shall be endorsed by the governing body and the medical director who are responsible for establishment and direction of the program and which indicates the staff person responsible for implementation of the pro- gram.

(c) The plan shall emphasize the ongoing nature of the quality assurance pro- gram and the comprehensiveness of the scope of the program which shall include monitoring and evaluation of the following:

(1)   Medical staff functions including:

(i)   Peer-based review of clinical performance of individuals with clinical privileges.

(ii)   Surgical case and tissue review. (2) Anesthesia   services. (3)   Nursing services.

(4)   Pharmaceutical services.

(5)   Pathology and radiology services. (6)   Infection   control procedures.

(7)   Procedures performed in the ASF and their necessity. (8) Reports of accidents, injuries and safety hazards.

(d) The plan shall include participation of practitioners and other health care personnel.

Source

The provisions of this § 557.2 amended October 22, 1999, effective November 22, 1999, 29 Pa.B. 5583. Immediately preceding text appears at serial page (256569).

§ 557.3. Quality Assurance and Improvement Program.

(a) The quality assurance program shall include monitoring and evaluation of data collected, based on defined criteria that reflect current knowledge and clinical experience and relate to the care provided by the service. Sources of data include the medical records, incident reports, infection control records and patient complaints. The medical record shall contain sufficient data to support the diagnosis and determine that the procedures are appropriate to the diagnosis. Facilities that treat pediatric patients shall segregate data regarding these patients.

(b) The quality assurance program shall provide for the identification of problems and actions taken—through the monitoring and evaluation process—which improve the quality of patient care.

(c) The frequency, severity and source of suspected problems or concerns are evaluated by practitioners and nurses.

(d) Measures shall be implemented to resolve important problems or concerns identified. The results of these corrective measures shall be monitored to assure that the problem has been satisfactorily resolved. Measures which may be taken include:

(1) Changes in policies and procedures. (2) Staffing   and assignment changes.

(3) Appropriate education and training. (4) Adjustments in clinical privileges.

(5)   Changes in equipment or physical plant.

(e) The program shall include a mechanism to assure that activities are documented and reports of the quality assurance activities are brought to the attention of the governing body. There shall be a periodic reappraisal of the program.

(f) The quality assurance program shall include the establishment of a quality assurance committee.

§ 557.4. Quality Assurance and Improvement Committee.

(a)   The Committee shall consist of the following:

(1)   A practitioner who is not an owner.

(2)   A representative of administration. (3)   A registered nurse.

(4)   Other health care personnel, as appropriate. (b) Committee functions shall include:

(1)   Evaluating data submitted as part of the quality assurance program. (2) Reviewing credentials.

(3)   Reviewing tissue examination reports. (4)   Reviewing infection control program.

(5)   Reviewing the standards of practice in all specific areas of the ASF. (c)   Committee records of the activities shall include:

(1)   Reports made to the governing body.

(2) Minutes of committee meetings including date, time, persons attending, description and results of cases reviewed and recommendations made by the committee.

(3) Corrective actions taken including appropriate orientation,

training or education programs necessary to correct deficiencies which are uncovered as a result of the quality assurance program.

Source

The provisions of this § 557.4 amended October 22, 1999, effective November 22, 1999, 29 Pa.B. 5583. Immediately preceding text appears at serial pages (256570) to (256571)

CHAPTER 559.

NURSING SERVICES

Authority

The provisions of this Chapter 559 issued under Chapter 8 of the Health Care Facilities Act (35 P. S. §§ 448.801a—448.820), specifically sections 448.801a and 448.803; and section 2102(a) and (g) of The Administrative Code of 1929 (71 P. S. § 532(a) and (g)), unless otherwise noted.

Source

The provisions of this Chapter 559 adopted January 23, 1987, effective March 25, 1987, 17 Pa.B. 376, unless otherwise noted.

§ 559.1. Nursing department.

The ASF shall have an organized nursing department under the supervision of a registered nurse who has responsibility and accountability for nursing services.

§ 559.2. Director of nursing.

The director of nursing shall be currently licensed as a registered nurse in this Commonwealth and be responsible and accountable to the person in charge of the ASF for:

(1) Delivery of nursing services to patients.

(2) Development and maintenance of nursing service goals and objectives, standards of nursing practice, nursing policy and procedure manuals and writ- ten job descriptions for each level of personnel.

(3) Coordination of nursing services with other patient services.

(4) Establishment of a means of assessing the nursing care needs of patients and staffing to meet those needs.

(5) Staff development.

Source

The provisions of this § 559.2 amended October 22, 1999, effective November 22, 1999, 29 Pa.B. 5583. Immediately preceding text appears at serial page (256573).

§ 559.3. Nursing personnel.

(a) An adequate number of licensed and assistive personnel shall be on duty to assure that staffing levels meet the total nursing needs of patients based on the number of patients in the facility and their individual nursing care needs. Class B and Class C ASFS which provide surgical services to pediatric patients shall have nursing staff with documented experience in the postoperative care of these patients.

(b) At least one registered nurse shall be in attendance during the hours patients are present. Nursing personnel shall be assigned to duties consistent with their education, training and experience.

(c) Registered professional nurses or licensed practical nurses practicing at an ASF shall be licensed to practice in this Commonwealth. There shall be a procedure to verify the licensure status of the nurses.

Source

The provisions of this § 559.3 amended October 22, 1999, effective November 22, 1999, 29 Pa.B. 5583. Immediately preceding text appears at serial pages (256573) to (256574).

§ 559.4. Staffing schedules.

(a) There shall be staffing schedules reflecting actual nursing personnel required for the ASF. Staffing patterns should reflect consideration of nursing goals, standards of nursing practice and the needs of the patients.

(b) Schedules which contain an indication of personnel attendance by date, and time of actual attendance shall be kept on file for a minimum of 1 year.

§ 559.5. Nursing notes.

Nursing notes shall be pertinent, accurate and concise so that they contribute to the continuity of patient care. Nursing records and reports shall become part of the patient's medical record.

CHAPTER 561.

PHARMACEUTICAL SERVICES

Authority

The provisions of this Chapter 561 issued under Chapter 8 of the Health Care Facilities Act (35 P. S. §§ 448.801a—448.820), specifically sections 448.801a and 448.803; and section 2102(a) and (g) of The Administrative Code of 1929 (71 P. S. § 532(a) and (g)), unless otherwise noted.

Source

The provisions of this Chapter 561 adopted January 23, 1987, effective March 25, 1987, 17 Pa.B. 376, unless otherwise noted.

GENERAL PROVISIONS

§ 561.1. Drugs and biologicals.

The ASF shall provide drugs and biologicals in a safe and effective manner to meet the needs of the patients and to adequately support the organization's clinical capabilities commensurate with their license classification, in accordance with accepted ethical and professional practice and applicable State and Federal law, including the Pharmacy Act (63 P. S. §§ 390.1—390.13), 49 Pa. Code Chapter 27 (relating to State Board of Pharmacy), The Controlled Substance, Drug, Device and Cosmetic Act (35 P. S. §§ 780-101—780-144) and Chapter 25 (relating to controlled substances, drugs, devices and cosmetics).

Source

The provisions of this § 561.1 amended October 22, 1999, effective November 22, 1999, 29 Pa.B. 5583. Immediately preceding text appears at serial page (256575).

§ 561.2. Pharmaceutical service.

(a) Pharmaceutical services shall be supervised by a physician or dentist who is qualified to assume professional, organization and administrative responsibility for the quality of services rendered. Practitioners may dispense drugs only to the patients who are in their care.

(b) A pharmacy owned and operated by the ASF shall be supervised by a licensed pharmacist.

(c) Contracted pharmaceutical services shall be provided in accordance with the same ethical and professional practices and legal requirements that would be required if these services are provided directly by the organization.

Source

The provisions of this § 561.2 amended October 22, 1999, effective November 22, 1999, 29 Pa.B. 5583. Immediately preceding text appears at serial page (256576).

PHARMACEUTICAL FACILITIES

§ 561.11. Principle.

The ASF shall provide equipment and supplies for the pharmaceutical service to implement its professional and administrative functions and to ensure patient safety through the proper storage and dispensing of drugs. Facilities shall be provided for the storage, safeguarding, preparation and dispensing of drugs.

§ 561.12. Supplies.

The pharmacist or practitioner in charge of the pharmaceutical service shall maintain a supply of drugs and devices adequate to meet the needs of the patients. Pharmacy supplies shall conform to 49 Pa. Code § 27.14 (relating to supplies).

§ 561.13. Storage.

The area in the ASF where drugs are stored shall be periodically checked by the responsible pharmacist or practitioner and proper logs maintained.

Source

The provisions of this § 561.13 amended October 22, 1999, effective November 22, 1999, 29 Pa.B. 5583. Immediately preceding text appears at serial page (256576).

§ 561.14. Space.

There shall be adequate space provided for pharmaceutical operations, and the storage of drugs at a satisfactory location provided with proper lighting. Ventilation and temperature controls shall be in accordance with 49 Pa. Code §§ 27.15 and 27.16 (relating to sanitary standards; and construction requirements).

§ 561.15. Locked storage.

Special locked storage space shall be provided to meet requirements for storage of controlled substances, alcohol and other prescribed drugs as set forth in Chapter 25 (relating to controlled substances, drugs, devices and cosmetics) and

49 Pa. Code §§ 27.16(b)(4) and 27.17 (relating to construction requirements; and security for Schedule II controlled substances).

POLICIES AND PROCEDURES

§ 561.21. Principle.

The scope of the pharmaceutical service shall be consistent with the medication needs of the patients and congruent with the license classification of the ASF. The pharmaceutical policies shall include a program for the control and account- ability of drug products throughout the ASF. If drugs are used for an experimental purpose, the use thereof shall be approved by an Institutional Review Board (IRB) or an IRB shall waive review and proper consent for use shall be obtained.

Source

The provisions of this § 561.21 amended October 22, 1999, effective November 22, 1999, 29 Pa.B. 5583. Immediately preceding text appears at serial page (256577).

§ 561.22. Records.

(a) Drug transactions of the pharmaceutical service shall be recorded, and those records shall be correlated with other ASF records. Records and security shall be maintained to assure the control and safe dispensing of drugs and compliance with Federal and Commonwealth statutes.

(b) Drugs ordered and administered to patients shall be documented in the medical record of the patient.

(c) Oral orders for drugs for immediate administration shall be followed by a written order, signed by the prescribing practitioner, prior to the discharge of the patient.

(d) Adverse drug reactions and drug sensitivities shall be recorded in the patient's medical record and copies maintained for review by the quality assurance committee.

§ 561.23. Use of controlled substances and other drugs.

There shall be policies and procedures developed and approved by the medical staff which establish controls governing the use of controlled substances and other drugs, including sedatives, anticoagulants, antibiotics, oxytoxics and corticosteroids. Policies shall be established regarding written orders for appropriate dosage of all drugs.

Source

The provisions of this § 561.23 amended October 22, 1999, effective November 22, 1999, 29 Pa.B. 5583. Immediately preceding text appears at serial page (256577).

§ 561.24. Emergency pharmaceutical services.

Provision shall be made for emergency pharmaceutical services. Emergency drugs shall be kept readily available and under the control of either the pharma- cist or the practitioner in charge of pharmaceutical services.

§ 561.25. Distressed drugs, devices and cosmetics.

Drugs, devices and cosmetics which are outdated, visibly deteriorated, unlabeled or inadequately labeled, recalled, discontinued or obsolete shall be identified by the licensed pharmacist or responsible practitioner and shall be disposed of in compliance with applicable Commonwealth and Federal regulations.

§ 561.26. Mishandling of drugs.

If there is reason to suspect mishandling of scheduled or controlled drugs, the person in charge of the ASF shall contact the Bureau of Drug Control of the Office of Attorney General or State or local police.

CHAPTER 563. MEDICAL RECORDS

Authority

The provisions of this Chapter 563 issued under Chapter 8 of the Health Care Facilities Act (35 P. S. §§ 448.801a—448.820), specifically sections 448.801a and 448.803; section 2101(a) and (g) of The Administrative Code of 1929 (71 P. S. § 532(a) and (g)), unless otherwise noted.

Source

The provisions of this Chapter adopted January 23, 1987, effective March 25, 1987, 17 Pa.B. 376, unless otherwise noted.

§ 563.1. Principle.

The ASF shall maintain complete, comprehensive and accurate medical records for every patient to ensure adequate patient care.

§ 563.2. Organization and staffing.

(a) The ASF shall have a medical record service. It shall be directed, staffed and equipped to ensure the accurate processing, indexing and filing of medical records.

(b) At least one full-time or part-time employee shall provide regular medical record service.

§ 563.3. Facilities.

The medical record service shall be properly equipped to enable its personnel to function in an effective manner and to maintain medical records so that they are readily accessible and secure from unauthorized use.

§ 563.4. Identification and filing of medical records.

The medical record service shall maintain a system of identification and filing to facilitate the prompt location of the medical record of a patient.

§ 563.5. Storage of medical records.

Medical records shall be stored to provide protection from loss, damage or unauthorized access.

§ 563.6. Preservation of medical records.

(a) The facility shall have a written policy regarding the retention of records. Medical records whether original, reproductions or microfilm, shall be kept on file for a minimum of 7 years following the discharge of a patient.

(b) If the patient is a minor, records shall be kept on file until his majority, and then, for 7 years or as long as the records of adult patients are maintained.

(c) If an ASF discontinues operation, it shall make known to the Department where its records are stored. Records are to be stored in a facility offering retrieval services for at least 5 years after the closure date. Prior to destruction, public notice shall be made to permit former patients or their representatives to claim their own records. Public notice shall be in at least two forms, legal notice and display advertisement in a local newspaper of general circulation.

§ 563.7. Microfilming medical records.

Medical records may be microfilmed at any time including immediately after completion. Microfilming may be done on or off the premises. If done off the premises, the ASF shall take precautions to assure the confidentiality and safe- keeping of the records. The original of microfilmed medical records may not be destroyed until the medical records service has had an opportunity to review the processed film for content.

§ 563.8. Automation or computerization of medical records.

Nothing in this subpart prohibits the use of automation or computerization in the medical records service, if the provisions in this chapter are met and the information is readily available for use in patient care. Innovations in medical record formats, compilation and data retrieval are specifically encouraged.

Source

The provisions of this § 563.8 amended October 22, 1999, effective November 22, 1999, 29 Pa.B. 5583. Immediately preceding text appears at serial page (256580).

§ 563.9. Confidentiality of medical records.

Records shall be treated as confidential. Only authorized personnel shall have access to the records. The written authorization of the patient shall be presented and then maintained in the original record as authority for release of medical information outside the ASF.

§ 563.10. Ownership.

There shall be written policies and procedures which specify who has access to medical records, under what conditions records may be removed from the ASF, and under what conditions medical record information may be released. Medical records are the property of the ASF, and they may not be removed from the premises except for court purposes. Copies may be made available for authorized appropriate purposes, such as insurance claims and practitioner review.

§ 563.11. Patient access.

Patients or patient designees shall be given access to or a copy of their medical records, or both. The patient or the patient's designee may be charged for the cost of reproducing the copies; however, the charges shall be reasonably related to the cost of making the copy.

§ 563.12. Form and content of record.

The ASF shall maintain a separate medical record for each patient. Every record shall be accurate, legible and promptly completed. Patient medical records shall be constructed to stand alone and be easily identified as ASF records. Medical records shall include at least the following:

(1)   Patient identification.

(2)   Pertinent medical history and results of physical examination.

(3)   Preoperative diagnostic studies—entered before surgery— if performed.

(4) The presence or absence of allergies and untoward drug reactions recorded in a prominent and uniform location in all patient charts on a current basis.

(5) Documentation of properly executed, informed patient consent. (6) Entries related to anesthesia administration.

(7) Findings and techniques of the operation, including a pathologist report on tissue removed during surgery.

(8) Notes by authorized staff members and individuals who have been granted clinical privileges, nurses' notes and entries by other professional personnel.

(9) Written and verbal disposition recommendations and instructions given to the patient.

(10) Significant medical advice given to a patient by telephone. (11) Discharge summary including discharge diagnosis.

Source

The provisions of this § 563.12 amended October 22, 1999, effective November 22, 1999, 29 Pa.B. 5583. Immediately preceding text appears at serial page (256581).

Cross References

This section cited in 28 Pa. Code § 563.13 (relating to entries).

§ 563.13. Entries.

(a) Entries in the record shall be dated and authenticated by the person making the entry.

(b) Symbols and abbreviations may be used only when they have been approved by the medical staff and when a legend exists to explain them.

(c) A single signature on the fact sheet of a record does not suffice to authenticate the entire record. Each entry shall be individually authenticated.

(d) Notation of unusual incidents shall be entered in the medical record.

(e) Necessary documentation on the patient's medical record as specified in

§ 563.12 (relating to form and content of record) shall be completed in a timely manner not to exceed 30 days.

Source

The provisions of this § 563.13 amended October 22, 1999, effective November 22, 1999, 29 Pa.B. 5583. Immediately preceding text appears at serial page (256581).

CHAPTER 565.

LABORATORY AND RADIOLOGY SERVICES

Authority

The provisions of this Chapter 565 issued under Chapter 8 of the Health Care Facilities Act (35 P. S. §§ 448.801a—448.820), specifically sections 448.801a and 448.803; section 2101(a) and (g) of The Administrative Code of 1929 (71 P. S. § 532(a) and (g)), unless otherwise noted.

Source

The provisions of this Chapter 565 adopted January 23, 1987, effective March 25, 1987, 17 Pa.B. 376, unless otherwise noted.

LABORATORY SERVICES

§ 565.1. Principle.

The ASF shall have procedures for obtaining routine and emergency laboratory services to meet the needs of patients.

§ 565.2. Laboratory service policy.

Laboratory services shall be provided under The Clinical Laboratory Act (35 P. S. §§ 2151—2165) and Chapter 5 (relating to clinical laboratories).

§ 565.3. Functions.

Laboratory functions shall include:

(1) Performing tests in a timely manner.

(2) Distributing test results within 24 hours after completion of a test and maintaining a copy of the results in the laboratory.

§ 565.4. Records.

Dated reports of services performed shall be made a part of the patient's medical record.

RADIOLOGY SERVICES

§ 565.11. Principle.

Radiology services provided or made available shall meet the needs of the patients and shall be provided in accordance with ethical and professional standards of the American Society of Radiologic

Technologists and the American College of Radiology.

§ 565.12. Radiology service policy.

(a) The service shall be provided by contract or directly by the ASF.

(b) Applicable provisions of the Department of Environmental Protection regulations in 25 Pa. Code Chapters 221—233 and 25 Pa. Code §§ 235.1 and235.11—235.15, and the United States Nuclear Regulatory Commission regulations in 10 CFR Chapter I (relating to Nuclear Regulatory Commission) shall be met by the ASF or its contracted radiology service.

Source

The provisions of this § 565.12 amended October 22, 1999, effective November 22, 1999, 29 Pa.B. 5583. Immediately preceding text appears at serial page (256584).

§ 565.13. Organization and staffing.

(a) Radiology services provided by the ASF shall be directed by a person who is qualified to assume professional, organizational and administrative responsibility for the quality of services rendered.

(b) Sufficient adequately trained, certified and experienced personnel shall be available to supervise and conduct the work of the radiology services.

Source

The provisions of this § 565.13 amended October 22, 1999, effective November 22, 1999, 29 Pa.B. 5583. Immediately preceding text appears at serial page (256584).

§ 565.14. Policies.

(a) Policies shall address the quality aspects of radiology services including, but not limited to:

(1) Performing radiology services only upon the written order of a practitioner, which shall be accompanied by a concise statement of the reason for the examination.

(2) Limiting the use of radioactive sources to qualified persons in the organization who have been granted privileges for the use on the basis of their training, experience and current competence.

(3) Storing and retaining of films.

(b) Policies shall address the safety aspects of radiology services including, but not limited to:

(1) Regulation of the use, removal, handling and storage of radioactive material.

(2) Precautions against electrical, mechanical and radiation hazards. (3) Proper shielding where radiation sources are used.

(4) Wearing of acceptable monitoring devices by personnel who might be exposed to radiation in an area with a radiation hazard.

(5) Maintenance of radiation exposure records on personnel.

(6) Instructions to personnel in safety precautions and in dealing with emergency radiation hazards.

(7) Periodic evaluation by qualified personnel of radiation sources and of safety measures followed, including calibration of equipment in compliance with Federal and Commonwealth statutes

and regulations and local ordinances. Authenticated, dated reports of services performed shall be made a part of the patient's medical record, in a timely manner not to exceed 30 days.

Source

The provisions of this § 565.15 amended October 22, 1999, effective November 22, 1999, 29 Pa.B. 5583. Immediately preceding text appears at serial page (256585).

§ 565.16. Facilities.

If radiology services are provided by the ASF, adequate space, equipment and supplies shall be provided to perform the volume of work with optimal accuracy, precision, efficiency and safety.

CHAPTER 567.

ENVIRONMENTAL SERVICES

Authority

The provisions of this Chapter 567 issued under Chapter 8 of the Health Care Facilities Act (35 P. S. §§ 448.801a—448.820), specifically sections 448.801a and 448.803; and section 2101(a) and (g)of The Administrative Code of 1929 (71 P. S. § 532(a) and (g)), unless otherwise noted.

Source

The provisions of this Chapter 567 adopted January 23, 1987, effective March 25, 1987, 17 Pa.B. 376, unless otherwise noted.

INFECTION CONTROL

§ 567.1. Principle.

The ASF shall have a sanitary environment, properly constructed, equipped and maintained to protect surgical patients and ASF personnel from cross-infection and to protect the health and safety of patients.

Source

The provisions of this § 567.1 amended October 22, 1999, effective November 22, 1999, 29 Pa.B. 5583. Immediately preceding text appears at serial page (256588).

§ 567.2. Committee responsibilities.

The quality assurance committee shall be responsible for:

(1) The prevention, control and investigation of infection in the ASF and for assuring the effectiveness of current procedural techniques in all departments.

(2) The designation of one full-time or one part-time employee responsible for developing and monitoring the infection control program including, but not limited to:

(i) Written standards for ASF sanitation and asepsis.

(ii) Procedures and techniques for meeting established sanitation and asepsis standards.

(iii) Isolation procedures.

(iv) Maintaining records of infections which originate in the ASF among patients and personnel to trace the sources of infection and to identify epidemic situations.

(v) Providing assistance in the development of the employee health pro- gram of the ASF.

(vi) Submitting a copy of pertinent findings and recommendations to the committee.

§ 567.3. Policies and procedures.

(a) Only authorized persons, who are properly attired, shall be allowed in the surgical area.

(b) Current written policies and procedures to assure definite and valid infection control shall include the following:

(1) Medical asepsis.

(2) Surgical asepsis.

(3) Sterilization and disinfection, including suitable equipment for routine and rapid sterilization.

(4) Sterilized materials are packaged, labeled and dated in a consistent manner.

(5) Housekeeping.

(6) Cleaning of surgical suites prior to each operation. (7) Clean and soiled linen and utility rooms.

(8) Linen.

(9) Traffic flow patterns. (10) Isolation protocols.

(11) Staff health status requirements.

(12) Infection control in-service education for personnel. (13) Recording and reporting of potential infection.

(14) Bacteriological testing of potential infections, recording results and reporting to the quality assurance committee.

(15) Admission criteria for patients with specific or suspected infections. (16) Patient postdischarge investigation.

(17) Reporting of communicable diseases as required by § 27.2 (relating to specific identified reportable diseases, infections and conditions).

Source

The provisions of this § 567.3 amended October 22, 1999, effective November 22, 1999, 29 Pa.B. 5583. Immediately preceding text appears at serial pages (256588) to (256589).

SUPPLIES

§ 567.11. Operating suite equipment.

The operating suite shall be adequately equipped with age appropriate equipment for the types of procedures to be performed and the recovery area shall be adequately equipped for the proper care of postanesthesia recovery of surgical patients. All equipment and supplies shall be age and size appropriate for the patients treated. The following equipment shall be available in the operating suite and recovery area.

(1) Suitable surgical instruments customarily available for the planned surgical procedure.

(2) Emergency call system.

(3)   Airways, breathing bag and device for the provision of positive pressure rescue breathing.

(4)   Cardio-pulmonary drugs and intubation equipment.

(5)   Cardiac monitor and defibrillator.

(6)   Resuscitator including oxygen and suction equipment.

(7)   Tracheostomy and necessary pulmonary reexpansion supplies.

Source

The provisions of this § 567.11 adopted January 23, 1987, effective March 25, 1987, 17 Pa.B. 376; amended July 21, 1989, effective July 22, 1989, 19 Pa.B. 3105; amended October 22, 1999, effective November 22, 1999, 29 Pa.B. 5583. Immediately preceding text appears at serial page (256589).

LINEN SERVICE

§ 567.21. Principle.

An adequate supply of clean linen, sterile linen and disposable materials shall be maintained.

§ 567.22. Linen service policy.

The ASF shall require the agency providing the linen service to maintain at least the standards outlined in this chapter, and the contract shall so state. The off-premises laundry service shall ensure that clean linen is completely packaged and is protected from contamination upon delivery to the ASF.

§ 567.23. Clean linen.

Clean linen shall be available to meet the daily and emergency needs of the ASF. Clean linen shall be handled and stored to minimize contamination from surface contact or airborne deposits.

§ 567.24. Soiled linen.

Soiled linen shall be collected and stored to avoid microbial dissemination into the environment. Soiled linen shall be kept segregated from clean linen. Soiled linen from isolation areas shall be identified and separately bagged. Precautions shall be taken in the subsequent processing of soiled linen from isolation areas to prevent microbial dissemination and infection.

HOUSEKEEPING SERVICES

§ 567.31. Principle.

The facility, the premises and equipment shall be kept clean and free of vermin, insects, rodents and litter.

§ 567.32. Policies and procedures.

Procedures shall be developed for cleaning and care of equipment, for establishment of cleaning schedules, for cleaning methods and for proper use of cleaning supplies and disposal of waste. Suitable equipment shall be provided to facilitate cleaning.

Source

The provisions of this § 567.32 amended October 22, 1999, effective November 22, 1999, 29 Pa.B. 5583. Immediately preceding text appears at serial page (256590).

§ 567.33. Waste disposal.

(a) Garbage shall be stored in tight, nonabsorbent and readily cleanable containers with tight-fitting lids. Garbage shall be removed from the premises as frequently as necessary to prevent nuisance and shall be disposed of in a manner consistent with Federal and Commonwealth regulations and local codes and ordinances.

(b) Refuse shall be stored in covered trash containers prior to removal.

(c) Pathological, bacteriological, surgical, gynecological and contaminated waste and similar materials shall be disposed of by a method approved by the Department of Environmental Resources under 25 Pa. Code Chapter 75 (relating to solid waste management) and in compliance with local ordinances.

MAINTENANCE SERVICE

§ 567.41. Principle.

The ASF shall be equipped, operated and maintained to sustain its safe and sanitary characteristics and to minimize health hazards in the ASF for the protection of patients and employees.

§ 567.42. Policies and procedures.

(a) A schedule of preventive maintenance shall be developed for the physical plant, biomedical and other equipment.

(b) Written procedures shall be readily available for employees to follow in the event of a breakdown in equipment, mechanical systems or utilities.

§ 567.43. Ventilation system.

The ventilation system shall be inspected and maintained in accordance with the written maintenance schedule to ensure that a properly conditioned air supply meeting minimum filtration, humidity and temperature requirements is provided in critical areas such as the surgical and recovery suites under Chapter 571 (relating to construction standards).

§ 567.51. Water supply.

MISCELLANEOUS

(a) Water shall be obtained from a municipal or private water system approved by the Department of Environmental Resources and in compliance with applicable Federal and Commonwealth regulations and local ordinances.

(b) Provisions shall be made for an emergency supply of water when the usual source of water is neither usable nor available.

§ 567.52. Lighting.

Glare-free artificial lighting shall be provided in all areas of the ASF. For cur- rent recommendations of lighting levels for ASFs, see the latest edition of the IES, (Illuminating Engineering Society), Lighting Handbook, Application Volume or Lighting for Health Care Facilities. Both documents are published by the IES of North America, 345 East 47th Street, New York, New York 10017.

§ 567.53. Sterilization control.

There shall be written policies to establish the following:

(1) A method of control to assure sterilization of supplies and water.

(2) Processing of sterile supplies at specified intervals.

(3) Use of disposable equipment.

CHAPTER 569.

FIRE AND SAFETY SERVICES

Authority

The provisions of this Chapter 569 issued under Chapter 8 of the Health Care Facilities Act (35 P. S. §§ 448.801a—448.820), specifically sections 448.801a and 448.803; and section 2102(a) and (g) of The Administrative Code of 1929 (71 P. S. § 532(a) and (g)), unless otherwise noted.

GENERAL PROVISIONS

§ 569.1. Principle.

The ASF shall have an organized fire, safety and disaster program under the direction and supervision of one or more persons qualified to implement the pro- gram.

§ 569.2. Fire safety standards.

(a) An ASF shall meet the applicable edition of National Fire Protection Association 101 Life Safety Code, which is currently adopted by the Department. (b) An ASF previously in compliance with prior editions of the Life Safety Code, is deemed in compliance with subsequent Life Safety Codes, except renovation or new construction shall meet the current edition adopted by the Department.

Source

The provisions of this § 569.2 amended October 22, 1999, effective November 22, 1999, 29 Pa.B. 5583. Immediately preceding text appears at serial page (256594).

Cross References

This section cited in 28 Pa. Code § 571.2 (relating to modifications to HHS requirements).

§ 569.3. Policies and procedures.

Written policies and procedures for use in preventing and responding to fire and disaster shall be available to personnel.

INTERNAL DISASTER PLAN

§ 569.11. Firefighting service.

The person in charge of the ASF shall establish a workable plan with the nearest fire department for fire- fighting service. The ASF shall provide the fire department with a current floor plan of the building showing the location of fire- fighting equipment, exits, patient rooms, storage places of flammable and information that the fire department requires or as may be necessary.

Source

The provisions of this § 569.11 amended October 22, 1999, effective November 22, 1999, 29 Pa.B. 5583. Immediately preceding text appears at serial page (256594).

§ 569.12. Fire warning and safety systems.

An ASF shall have an automatic and manually activated fire alarm system installed to transmit an alarm automatically to the fire department by the most direct and reliable method approved by local ordinances.

§ 569.13. Testing fire warning systems.

Fire safety systems, including automatic fire extinguishing systems, automatic and manual alarms, stand-pipes and hose reels shall be of an approved type. They shall be kept in good operating condition and inspected by qualified ASF personnel at least every 3 months. Records of the inspections shall be kept on file for the licensure period.

§ 569.14. Internal disaster and fire plans.

The ASF shall have an internal disaster and fire plan incorporating evacuation procedures and the safety of both closed records and the records of those patients being evacuated. These plans shall be made available to personnel and evacuation diagrams shall be posted throughout the ASF.

§ 569.15. Safety education program.

Employees shall participate in the safety program and perform the duties delegated to them and be instructed in the operation of the fire warning system, the proper use of fire fighting equipment and the procedure to follow if electric power is impaired.

§ 569.21. Fire drills.

EVACUATION DRILLS

(a) Fire, internal disaster and evacuation drills shall be held at least quarterly for ASF personnel and under varied conditions.

(b) The CEO shall:

(1) Ensure that all personnel are trained to perform assigned duties.

(2) Ensure that all personnel are familiar with the use and operation of the firefighting equipment in the ASF.

(3) Enable the chief executive officer to evaluate the effectiveness of the plan.

(c) A written report and evaluation of drills conducted since the last survey shall be kept on file.

(d) The actual evacuation of patients to safe areas during a drill is optional.

Source

The provisions of this § 569.21 amended October 22, 1999, effective November 22, 1999, 29 Pa.B. 5583. Immediately preceding text appears at serial page (256595).

SAFETY PRECAUTIONS

§ 569.31. Emergency power.

The emergency electric power source and associated equipment shall be regularly inspected, tested and maintained in accordance with current NFPA Standards. A written record shall be maintained of inspection, performance, exercising period and repairs of emergency power equipment

§ 569.32. Fire inspection.

The ASF shall request an annual inspection by its local fire department.

§ 569.33. Smoking.

Smoking is not permitted in an ASF.

Source

The provisions of this § 569.33 amended October 22, 1999, effective November 22, 1999, 29 Pa.B. 5583. Immediately preceding text appears at serial page (256596).

§ 569.34. Electrical safety.

Appliances, instruments and installations shall be tested before use to deter- mine compliance with grounding, current leakage and other device safety requirements to ensure protection of patients and employees. A program of routine maintenance shall be effectively enforced to ensure that electrical receptacles and plugs, wires and connectors are safe. If an appliance requiring three-wire circuitry for grounding is attached to a two-wire outlet, the adaptor plug pigtail shall be attached to a ground.

§ 569.35. General safety precautions.

The following safety precautions shall be met:

(1) Doorways, corridors and stairwells shall be properly lighted and free of obstructions.

(2) Doors into patient rooms may not be locked.

(3) Exit doors may not be locked from the inside while patients are in the ASF.

(4) Doors opening to shafts shall be equipped with self-closing devices and positive latches.

(5) Wastebaskets, cubicle curtains, window shades and drapes shall be rendered flame retardant.

(6) Call bells in the shower, tub room or water closet shall be easily accessible to patients.

(7) Only nonflammable agents may be present in a surgical suite.

Source

The provisions of this § 569.35 amended October 22, 1999, effective November 22, 1999, 29 Pa.B. 5583. Immediately preceding text appears at serial page (256596).

§ 569.36. Safety devices.

The following safety devices shall be provided:

(1) Grab bars within reaching distance on at least one side of toilets, bathtubs and showers used by patients.

(2) Bedside rails on both sides of a bed for use when the condition of the patient warrants.

§ 569.37. Report of emergencies causing interruption of service.

(a) The person in charge of the ASF shall make a report of any emergency, such as a strike, fire or natural disaster which significantly interrupts or alters ASF services and threatens the health and safety of patients, and which requires one of the following:

(1) The services of a fire department.

(2) The evacuation of a patient.

(3) The use of nonmedical emergency equipment.

(b) The report made under subsection (a) shall be submitted to the Director of the Division of Hospitals of the Department as soon as possible, and shall include the following information:

(1) Time, date, cause, location and nature of emergency. (2) Number of patients evacuated.

(3) Loss of life and name of a deceased patient.

(4) Names of patients sent to other facilities and names of the facilities.

(5) Assistance required from the Health Department to protect the health and safety of the patients.

(c) Oral reports shall be followed by a complete written report verifying the information in subsection (b). The written report shall be dated and shall be authenticated by the person in charge.

CHAPTER 571.

CONSTRUCTION STANDARDS

Authority

The provisions of this Chapter 571 issued under Chapter 8 of the Health Care Facilities Act (35 P. S. §§ 448.801a—448.820), specifically sections 448.801a and 448.803; and section 2102(a) and (g) of The Administrative Code of 1929 (71 P. S. § 532(a) and (g)), unless otherwise noted.

Source

The provisions of this Chapter 571 adopted January 23, 1987, effective March 25, 1987, 17 Pa.B. 376, unless otherwise noted.

Cross References

This chapter cited in 28 Pa. Code § 567.43 (relating to ventilation system).

GENERAL PROVISIONS

§ 571.1. Minimum standards.

ASF construction shall be in accordance with the latest edition of the "Guide- lines for Design and Construction of Hospital and Health Care Facilities," as published by the American Institute of Architects/Academy of Architecture for Health including those guidelines established for various outpatient facilities. In the alternative, a facility shall meet the construction guidelines for specified types of surgical procedures as listed in Appendix A (relating to alternative construction guidelines). Where renovation or replacement work is performed within an existing facility, all new work or additions shall comply with the requirements for new construction.

Source

The provisions of this § 571.1 amended October 22, 1999, effective November 22, 1999, 29 Pa.B. 5583. Immediately preceding text appears at serial page (256599).

§ 571.2. Modifications to HHS requirements.

(a) Life Safety Code means the standard as defined in § 569.2 (relating to fire safety standards).

(b) Adequate storage areas shall be provided to meet the needs of the facility.

(c) Patient privacy shall be provided in preoperative and postoperative areas.

(d) In multistory buildings, where the ASF may be provided on floors other than at grade level, at least one hospital type elevator shall be provided.

(e) Elevators shall conform to "HHS Requirements" and the latest edition of the "American National Standard Safety Code for Elevators, Dumbwaiters, Escalators and Moving Stairs."

(f) The Americans with Disabilities Act of 1990 (ADA) (42 U.S.C.A. §§ 12101−12213).

Source

The provisions of this § 571.2 amended October 22, 1999, effective November 22, 1999, 29 Pa.B. 5583. Immediately preceding text appears at serial page (256600).

SUBMISSION OF PLANS

§ 571.11. Principle.

Plans and specifications shall be submitted to the Division of Safety Inspection of the Department for approval prior to construction of an ASF, in accordance with § 51.5 (relating to building occupancy). Submission shall be in three stages.

Source

The provisions of this § 571.11 amended October 22, 1999, effective November 22, 1999, 29 Pa.B. 5583. Immediately preceding text appears at serial page (256600).

§ 571.12. Submission stages.

(a) First stage. One copy of the narrative description and one copy of the schematic drawings shall be provided.

(1) Program narrative.

(i) List in outline form the rooms or spaces to be included in each department, explaining the functions or services to be provided in each, indicating the approximate size, the number of personnel and the kind of equipment or furniture it will contain. Note special or unusual services or equipment to be included in the facility.

(ii)   Give an outline of construction materials.

(2)   Schematic plans.

(i) Single line drawings of each floor shall show the relationship of the various departments or services to each other and the room arrangement in each department. The name of each room shall be noted. The proposed roads and walks, service and entrance courts, parking and orientation may be shown on either a small plot plan or the first floor plan. A simple vertical space diagram shall be submitted at this stage.

(ii) If the project is an addition or is otherwise related to existing buildings on the site, the plans shall show the facilities and general arrangement of those buildings.

(b) Second stage. Two copies of the preliminary plans shall be provided. (1) Architectural.

(i) One-eighth inch scale floor plans of basement, floors and roof showing space assignment, sizes and outline of fixed and movable equipment.

(ii) Elevations and typical wall sections.

(iii) Plot plan showing roads, parking and sidewalks.

(2) Mechanical.

(i) Single line layouts of duct and piping systems which include air rates for determining pressure relationships.

(ii)   Riser diagrams for multi-story construction. (3)   Electrical.

(i)   Plans showing space assignment, sizes and outline of fixed equipment, such as transformers, main switch and switchboards and generator sets. (ii)   Simple riser diagram for multi-story building construction showing arrangement of feeders, subfeeders, bus work, load centers and branch circuit panels.

(c) Third stage—contract documents. Four sets of drawings shall be pro- vided, complete and adequate for bid contract and construction purposes. Drawings shall be prepared for each of the following branches of work: architectural, structural, mechanical and electrical.

(1) Drawings may be no less than 1/8 inch scale and show indications of fixed and movable equipment.

(2) If necessary, 1/4 inch scale drawing shall be included.

(3) Fire-rated assemblies, such as U.L., Factory Mutual and the like—shall be included on the drawings.

(4) Specifications shall supplement the drawings to fully describe the types, sizes, capacities, workmanship, finishes and other characteristics of materials and equipment.

§ 571.13. [Reserved].

Source

The provisions of this § 571.13 reserved October 22, 1999, effective November 22, 1999, 29 Pa.B. 5583. Immediately preceding text appears at serial page (256601).

APPENDIX A. ALTERNATIVE CONSTRUCTION GUIDELINES

ENDOSCOPY

1) Office Endoscopy, edited by Bergein F. Overholt and Sarkis J. Chobanian.

2) Planning an Endoscopy Suite for Office and Hospital, by Jerome D. Waye and Martin E. Rich.

Source

The provisions of this Appendix A adopted October 22, 1999, effective November 22, 1999, 29 Pa.B. 5583.

CHAPTER 573. [Reserved]

§§ 573.1 and 573.2.

[Reserved].

Source

The provisions of these §§ 573.1 and 573.2 adopted January 23, 1987, effective March 25, 1987, 17 Pa.B. 376; reserved October 22, 1999, effective November 22, 1999, 29 Pa.B. 5583. Immediately preceding text appears at serial pages (256603) to (256604).

There are is wealth of information on the internet that you can use to obtain additional information in your role as a board member. Your administrative team should be accessing these sites on a regular basis. For your information, we have provided the following links for you to review research on your own:

CMS Web Site

The CMS web site provides a considerable amount of information about your Medicare certification. Here are links to important information available:

Ambulatory Surgery Center Portal:

https://www.cms.gov/Center/Provider-Type/Ambulatory-Surgical-Centers-ASC-Center.html

Medicare Payment Information:

https://www.cms.gov/Medicare/Medicare-Fee-for-Service-Payment/ASCPayment/index.html

ASC Association

The Ambulatory Surgery Center Association is a nonprofit association that represents all aspects of the Ambulatory Surgery Center industry including the physicians, nurses, administrative staff and owners. The web site provides access to information about all aspects about the industry:

www.ascassociation.org

National Fire Protection Association (NFPA)

According to the NFPA website at www.nfpa.org, "the association delivers information and knowledge through more than 300 consensus codes and standards, research, training, education, outreach and advocacy; and by partnering with others who share an interest in furthering the NFPA mission." All NFPA codes and standards can be viewed on their website for free. To print the standards, you will have to purchase access. You can also buy copies of the published books either through NFPA or an online bookseller.

Note that as of the date of publication of this book, CMS has adopted the 2000 Edition of NFPA 101. It is expected that shortly, CMS will adopt the 2012 Edition.

Association for Professionals in Infection Control and Epidemiology (APIC)

APIC (www.apic.org) is one of the leading sources of infection control standards for the ASC industry. The organization publishes various books and provides regular training programs on infection control.

APIC provides regular training for infection control coordinators in ASCs and it has become the "defacto" standard that these coordinators attend this course.

Association for Operating Room Nurses (AORN)

AORN (www.aorn.org) is one of the most influential societies in the ASC industries and ASCs should encourage operating room staff members to join the organization and become CNOR Certified (Certified Nurse Operating Room).

AORN publishes a variety of books that provide guidance and standards for operating room management. Their educational programs provide training in a variety of areas applicable to ambulatory surgery centers.

Their publication "Guidelines for Perioperative Practice" is the industry's leading guide for operating room standards. Every ASC should maintain a copy of this book.

Certified Ambulatory Surgery Center Credential (CASC)

The CASC credential is overseen by the Board of Ambulatory Surgery Certification (www.aboutcasc.org). Administrators and nursing directors who wish to obtain the CASC credential must undergo a rigorous test to determine their knowledge of the industry and the responsibilities of the chief executive officer of ASCs.

To reduce the risk that the organization hires unqualified individuals, your governing bodies may wish to consider hiring administrators that carry the CASC credential.

The Facility Guidelines Institute (FGI)

FGI provides information about the *Guidelines for Design and Construction Health Care Facilities* – the definitive guide for construction standards applicable to healthcare organizations, including ambulatory surgery centers. The web site provides information about the guidelines and links to purchase the official books. Their web site is:

http://www.fgiguidelines.org/index.php

Eden Group Development, Inc.

The publisher of this book and the author maintain a web site where you can purchase books specifically written for the ambulatory surgery center industry at;

http://www.reg-books.com

The books include the best-selling The Survey Guide for ASCs - A Guide to the CMS Conditions for Coverage & Interpretive Guidelines for Ambulatory Surgery Centers and Ambulatory Surgery Center Governance - A Guide for Ambulatory Surgery Center Owners & Governing Body Members. These books are important additions to your ASC library and will help you prepare for a survey.

Ambulatory Healthcare Strategies, LLC

The author is also a nationally known consultant and maintains a web site at:

http://www.ah-strategies.com

Ambulatory Healthcare Strategies, LLC (AHS) caters to the Ambulatory Surgery (ASC) and Office-Based Surgery industry. AHS provides a full range of services to meet the administrative, regulatory and financial needs of your organization. AHS is NOT a management company, but provides many of the same services that a traditional management company provides. AHS don't take ownership, and their on-going fees are on a retainer basis with a fixed monthly fee.

Ambulatory Healthcare Strategies provides a unique business model – totally focused on what your organization's needs – not on a "cookie cutter" approach to outsourced services. Their business model provides a variety of outsourced service offerings ranging from one-time consulting services up to on-going retainer-based oversight services.

The AHS monthly fixed retainer-based Regulatory & Accreditation Oversight and Financial Oversight Services are unique to the industry and can often replace existing management company services for a fraction of the cost.

AHS Consulting Services include:

- Responding to State, CMS and Accreditation Surveys (Plan of Correction, Mitigation of Citations, Crisis Management)
- Interim Administrator/Clinical Management Services
- Accreditation and CMS Survey Preparation and Mock Surveys
- Financial Projections and Feasibility Studies
- Policy & Procedure Review and Updates and Maintenance Services
- Business Office, Billing System and Billing Service Reviews

Monthly Retainer Services:

Retainer services are geared specifically to the needs of your organization and the monthly fixed retainer fee is based on the services that you request. AHS does not require long-term contracts and their low overhead assures our fees are considerably less than the same services provided by a management company.

Owners and administrators of surgery centers and office based surgery practices major challenge in keeping up with the constant changes in the regulatory environment. Their retainer services are designed to give you the information and resources you need to keep current – without having to hire full-time compliance staff.

AHS monthly retainers can include:

- Maintenance of your Policy and Procedure Manual
- Oversight of your QI Program
- Attendance at your Committee and Governing Body Meetings and preparation of the agenda and minutes
- Preparation and management of your organizations strategic plan and goals and objectives
- Preparation of Monthly and Quarterly Financial Statements
- Assistance in preparing QI Studies
- State and Federal Reporting
- On-site training and education
- Preparation of budgets and financial projections
- Assistance in ownership transfers and recruitment
- Negotiations of Contracts
- Credentialing and Employee File oversight and electronic file maintenance
- Attendance at Surveys and preparation for upcoming surveys, follow-up after surveys

All retainers include:

- Access to the Surgery Center Academy – an on-line training portal providing employee orientation and annual mandatory education programs prepared specifically for your organization. This can supplement and or replace many of your in-house training programs

- Access to our unique database of educational programs for administrators and managers in your organization
- Annual Mock Survey for compliance with CMS Conditions for Coverage
- On-going text, email and phone access to our staff 24/7.

For more information, visit the AHS web site at www.ah-strategies.com or call John Goehle directly at 585-594-1167.

John J. Goehle is the Chief Operating Officer and partner with Ambulatory Healthcare Strategies, LLC based in Rochester, New York.

John is a Certified Public Accountant licensed in the State of New York and holds a Master's in Business Administration from Heriot-Watt University in Edinburgh, Scotland. He also holds the prestigious Certified Administrator – ASC (CASC) credential.

John is a 27 year veteran of ambulatory surgery centers and a national leader in ASC industry. He is a popular speaker on ASC finance, accounting, budgeting and administration. He has taught college courses in health care finance, economics and information systems. In 2005 he wrote "Finance Management Made Easy – Strategies for Ambulatory Surgery Centers" for HC Pro. In 2008 he wrote "APCs for ASCs Strategies for Success Under the New Payment System", also for HC Pro. He also co-authored both the first and second editions of the ASC Association's (formerly FASA) book "Finance and Accounting for ASC's."

You may contact the author through email at jgoehle@ah-strategies.com.

www.ingramcontent.com/pod-product-compliance
Lightning Source LLC
Chambersburg PA
CBHW071257220526
45468CB00001B/171